Resounding praise for

Hope in a Dark Tunnel

Your roadmap to well-being when navigating chronic illness

By Bev Roberts

"A practical and inspirational whole-self guide to getting your life back!"

~ Deanna Minich, PhD, *author of* The Rainbow Diet

"Masterfully structured, *'Hope in a Dark Tunnel'* provides just that and then some. Bev Roberts speaks from, and to, the heart in chronicling her trying journey through the shadows of chronic illness so that others might be saved unnecessary pain. It's a must-read and matchless reference companion for anyone in, or connected to, that struggle."

~ Dr. Bridget Cooper, *bestselling author of* Pain Rebel and Little Landslides

I would like to congratulate Bev Roberts on writing her book *'Hope in a Dark Tunnel'*! It is a story about a real person going through a real life challenge. Stories like this are always powerful in giving others hope and a resolve to face their own problems. But this book gives the reader more than hope, it outlines a path to follow. A path leading to not only recovery from physical illness, but to dealing with life's challenges as a whole. I warmly recommend it!

~ Dr Natasha Campbell-McBride, MD, *bestselling author of* Gut and Psychology Syndrome

Bev has created a brilliant roadmap for those with chronic debilitating illness to find their way out of the Dark Tunnel of despair, and to rebuild a life of hope and health one do-able step at a time. Both simple steps and complex processes are laid out in a way that allows the ill and their carers to work their way through from despair to triumph over adversity. It is a must-read for everyone touched by chronic health problems

~ Dr Mark Donohoe, MB BS FASLM

Bev's journey is unfortunately common, and yet so often hidden as those suffering are dismissed, shamed and blamed—especially when their illness is not visible. *'Hope in a Dark Tunnel'* seeks to upend all of that by empowering you to advocate for your own wellness, be in touch with your body, and provide it the compassion and help it needs to be well. *'Hope in a Dark Tunnel'* is full of very practical guidance taken step by step so you can apply it as you work through health challenges or just seek wellness more broadly in your life. As Bev puts it so beautifully, it lets you "see yourself as a well being."

~ Bryan Falchuk, *bestselling author of* Do a Day:
How to live a better life every day

"If you are one of the millions of people struggling with chronic illness with no relief in sight, let Bev be your guide back to hope. She's been where you are, and she has the know-how and actionable steps you need to experience better health and well-being. As you read through this book, you'll get to know Bev as a good friend and support system who can help you make it through this challenging time in your life."

~ Andrea Beaman, Holistic Health Coach
and Herbalist

There is much wisdom and depth in this relatively short book. It tells of the author's journey from relative wellness to illness and dis-ease and back again. If anyone is suffering physically, mentally or even spiritually, read it. If a friend or family member is not firing on all cylinders, read it. If you are just OK and want to stay well, read it too. It's a story and message bravely shared which deserves to reach a wide audience.

~ Tom Evans, Insight Timer meditation guide and co-author of The Big Ü

Chronic illness is the pits. It's invisible and nearly always isolating. People tend to comment on how you look without any enquiry about how you feel. If you have a chronic illness, you're going to love this book. Not only has it been written by someone who's walked the journey back to radiant health, but Bev is incredibly knowledgeable and shares what she's learned so you don't have to search for information that's helpful to your recovery. You'll find yourself dipping in and out of '*Hope in a Dark Tunnel*' as it will become your new best friend!

~ Petrea King, author of Up Until Now

Hope in a Dark Tunnel

Your roadmap to well-being when
navigating chronic illness

Bev Roberts

Copyright © 2018 by Bev Roberts
www.livingfabulously.com
email: hello@livingfabulously.com

Published by Bev Roberts, Sydney, Australia

Cover design: Karen Gunton
Art work: Julie Gibbons

For Alexis and Evelyn
You are the bright rainbow in any cloud

Contents

Introduction

*Resilience isn't developed by distraction from unwanted feelings,
but by realising that you can only thrive when you
travel through the pain of life's challenges.*
Jarl Forsman and Steve Sekhon

Are you facing a chronic health challenge and have
conflicting, or just too much information on how to
improve but still aren't sure where to begin?

I share the information in this book with you because I
don't want you to have to go through what I went through;
the merry-go-round of tests, doctors and the general feelings
of doubt and invisibility.

This book enables you to appreciate how much progress you
can make in managing your well-being and helps you
recognise the opportunities that are available to you.

You will feel understood and supported to take back your
personal power by

- **Getting back to basics**: Nurture yourself with
  goodness by eating well, sleeping well, moving more
  and increasing your self-care;
- **Managing your mindset**: Clean up your self-talk,
  focus on what you can do, show gratitude for simple
  pleasures and use realistic ways of measuring
  progress; and
- **Gaining knowledge**: Explore your chronic health
  challenges with an open mind and examine treatment
  options available while factoring in your own needs.

I want to ensure that you don't feel alone on the journey back to well-being and do not need to be defined by your chronic illness. We'll get to the heart of the matter by

- Recognising what you need to do to support yourself physically, mentally, emotionally and soulfully,
- Nourishing your body, mind and soul with consistency not perfection, learning to trust yourself along the way,
- Raising your awareness about the way relationships change when you get sick,
- Understanding why it's important to surround yourself with supportive people, and
- Acknowledging why it's equally important to pull back from non-supportive people.

Throughout the book you will find I use the hyphenated word 'well-being' as if they were two words. This is intentional because we will not only be exploring how you can take back your personal power and be resilient, but how you can truly become a well being.

This is not to dismiss that you are experiencing chronic health challenges or an invisible chronic illness. However, I do want to highlight that your physical, mental, emotional and soulful aspects are integrated, and it is important that you are able to take all these aspects into account so that you can see yourself as a well being.

I have also purposely chosen to use the word 'need' throughout the book. I am making a distinction between

Need: something you must have, and
Want: something you would like to have.

I know how easy it is to go into victim mode. It can feel as if it's easier to take the path of least resistance when you're dealing with a debilitating chronic health challenge that's difficult to diagnose or treat. For myself, doing that initially cost me many expensive tests and ineffective treatments, plus a lot of uncertainty and pain.

I'm certain that it's worth putting in the effort to become your own well-being champion and advocate. I know, as well as anyone, how difficult it can be to get out of our comfort zones, but I wouldn't go back to that feeling of helplessness and disempowerment either. My journey has me living more fabulously each new day, and that's my wish for you.

And if you are a carer or health professional, I want to help you gain a better understanding of how an invisible chronic illness feels from the patient's perspective.

My journey here

*Our journey through life is short. The wise know that even
though we can't control events or how long we're here,
we do get to choose how we interpret what happens.*
Jarl Forsman and Steve Sekhon

I have a strong work ethic and used to work hard and play
hard. I was passionate about achieving. As an award-winning
and board-certified executive, I worked sixty-plus hour
weeks and even in my own consulting business, I worked
extended hours.

I was unable to switch off from work. I was constantly
pushing myself to do the best I could for my family and for
the clients and colleagues I worked with.

I did not place a priority on myself or my capacity to take
time out. I was a human doing – not a human being – and it
took a great toll on my health, well-being and my
relationships. Quite simply, it sucked the joy out of my life.

Working so hard ensured I was out of touch with my body
and my emotions, I didn't have time to take stock of myself.
The many physical symptoms (joint pain, rashes, ice-pick
headaches) I began to experience seemed unrelated, so I put
up with them and soldiered on for six months.

The worst of the symptoms (poor memory recall, inability to
make decisions, lack of focus) were not related to my
physical body but to the chronic fatigue, brain fog and the
impaired way that my brain was functioning.

I finally realised that I was more than *just* exhausted. However, it took me a long time to accept that I was extremely ill.

Losing my mind

I found myself forgetting essential information on a regular basis. I forgot the names of people I worked with. I would stare at objects in my home and not know what to call them. There were times when I had wanted to say something, but the words would not come out my mouth. It felt as if there was a disconnect between my brain and my speech. I felt so frightened and traumatised by not being able to recall things I knew.

The reckoning point was when my daughter got frustrated with me for repeating the same statement or asking questions over and over within a short timeframe.

I had previously completed a Master's Degree in Behavioural Change and strategy while working full time as an executive. So, I felt distraught when I could not comprehend and interpret what I was reading, not even a paragraph in a women's magazine.

The joy of rest

I made the decision to take a three-month sabbatical. Part of me rationalised that I was burned out and if I were to rest and relax, I would feel my usual bouncy self again.

I chose to go to Italy where they're known for their ability to live the good life, where rest is a part of daily life and Sundays are sacred. My new mantra was "la dolce far niente" - the "sweetness of doing nothing" - a phrase made mainstream by Elizabeth Gilbert in *Eat, Pray, Love*. I was going to learn the art of living.

I lived like a local, got fresh produce from the markets and created a slow, gentle rhythm to each day. In southern Italy I learned to relish a 'siesta', as between 2pm and 5pm nothing is open, so it was completely acceptable to rest, and I knew I wouldn't miss out on anything. I continued this approach as I travelled into France.

By sleeping a lot, nurturing myself with whole, nutritious food, gentle walking and lots of rest, I began to feel a bit better, which reinforced my belief that my impairments were *just* caused by exhaustion.

Back to reality

After a conversation with a girlfriend in the United Kingdom, I realised that I was not ready to return to Australia. She invited me to stay in the Kent countryside, where I spent a month slowly re-integrating into daily life with her young family, while still taking life at a snail's pace.

On my return I felt optimistic. I recall going into my functional medicine doctor's office when I got back from my sabbatical saying how much better I felt compared to four months prior. Unfortunately, it was transitory.

A colleague of mine and I worked together for two days as co-facilitators for a leadership team event and I was unable to get out of bed for a few days afterwards.

I also went back to my personal trainer to resume my exercise routine, but the exertion made me so fatigued that my 'siesta' started as early as 10am and often repeated during the day.

A welcome input

It had been ten months since I'd gotten so ill and it was clear to me in those first couple of weeks back from travelling that things were not as they needed to be with my health and well-being.

I had taken four months off and yet two months later I was still not in the space to be able to seek consulting work. I couldn't continue with the status quo and I couldn't sustain the cost base I had with my savings.

I didn't know where to turn. I was self-employed so couldn't get support from an organisation. I contacted my financial broker and asked if I had any insurance that would help in the short-term. He confirmed that I did have income protection cover and that I was eligible to claim it. This was a real turning point in my journey. I have never had to be so resilient and stand so firmly in my truth as I did in the negative experiences that were to come.

Unexpected responses

As you may not know me, I will share that I am highly principled and hold myself accountable to my inner compass. I am known for my integrity and trustworthiness in business and personal interactions.

However, in their independent medical evaluations for the insurer, I was painted by a rheumatologist and a forensic psychiatrist as a post-menopausal, overweight hypochondriac who was feigning illness.

The pain of not being believed was immense and added more stress to an already distressing situation. I felt the weight of hopelessness bear down on me. It felt as if I was in a dark tunnel without any hope of getting the support I needed; there was no light at the end, or anywhere else I could see. I felt completely overwhelmed.

A neuropsychological independent medical evaluation was then requested to establish whether I was feigning / exaggerating symptoms or whether I was suffering from a genuine disorder.

During the assessment, the neuro-psychologist kept asking if I wanted to return another day as it took me six hours instead of her estimated three hours to complete the cognitive function tests.

I wanted to give up many times during those six hours. Taking frequent breaks outside in the fresh air and thinking about the imminent birth of my first granddaughter kept me going.

The report of my results noted the presence of cortical dysfunction (i.e. there does appear to be an illness present - it's just unclear what this happens to be). And I have to say, the relief I felt was indescribable. I was no longer perceived as a malingerer and hypochondriac.

It was only after this report that I was assigned to a support team, nine months after lodging my claim. I am so grateful to the psychologist assigned to my case. She gave me encouragement and created several opportunities for remediation and support.

However, as I was starting to feel supported by the insurer, I began facing challenges from an unexpected quarter of my life. Some of my family and friends didn't seem to understand or accept that I was ill.

Perhaps this was because most of my life I'd been the 'strong one' or the one people said would never retire because I was too busy all the time.

It was incredibly hurtful, and I felt so unsupported. I began to question and doubt myself again. I know the mind and body have a strong connection. However, I knew that this wasn't about my mental health. I knew I was dealing with something more.

What I came to realise is that if you have no diagnosis or an invisible chronic illness, it can be hard for people to understand where you're at. People are often misinformed about illnesses that they can't see physical manifestations of, such as chronic fatigue syndrome or fibromyalgia.

In time I learned to have compassion for their position. I realised that it was more about them and their perspective than about their response being a personal affront towards me.

My functional medicine doctor suggested that when people asked me how I was, I didn't give them any information about the state of my health. Instead, I would say that I was taking small steps in the right direction and leave it at that. It certainly helped.

Surrendering to what was

After one of the many very expensive tests, the results were clear that biotoxin illness was a contributing factor. Dr Ritchie Shoemaker describes biotoxin illness as "an acute and chronic, systemic inflammatory response syndrome acquired following exposure to the interior environment of a water-damaged building". The apartment I was living in had been gutted by fire and refurbished before I moved in. When the practitioner reviewed my results, her recommendation was to move out of my apartment immediately.

I felt so overwhelmed because I had nowhere to go that had no visible mould, carpets or curtains. When I shared this with two of my girlfriends they amazingly offered for me to stay with them.

It was a big step for me to surrender to what my reality was and to accept help from other people. I will be forever grateful for those two girlfriends, who took me in unconditionally and supported me in the next steps of my journey.

Retraining my brain

As an accredited change manager master, I have a deep interest in neuroscience and the plasticity of the brain. I've been a lifelong student and I love learning, so this seemed a natural way to rebuild my brain and recreate neural pathways for things that I'd taken for granted but had lost along the way.

I explored some learning opportunities to help myself, and others, and I quickly realised that this might also help me build an income stream. As I'd spent more than twenty-five years in corporate mentoring and coaching people, the best fit for me was to retrain as a well-being coach.

I found a course that I was able to take that supported learning by repetition, it gave small chunks of information at a time and I could listen to video lectures at my own pace.

Being able to take notes by hand supported the creation of new neural pathways for my brain.

Having an accountability buddy in my peer group to discuss content with and make meaning of was invaluable. I am proud to say that I passed each assessment and in twelve months I gained my certification as an integrative and holistic well-being coach.

Life is different

It's taken time, but I've learned to ask for help from people when I need it. I was genuinely surprised at how willing people are to help when you ask. It's not something I had done before as I'd been so self-reliant.

My busy social life was completely impacted by my chronic illness because I no longer had the 'get up and go' to get up and play. If it weren't for some good friends, I would have been isolated.

They were remarkable. They met me where I was and with what I was capable of doing, even if it only meant a short phone call to chat or a shared lunch at home.

Beyond my control

One of the biggest lessons I've learned on this journey has been that I don't need to control everything in my life. Previously, I had been over scheduled, overly busy, with very little time for spontaneity and time to be me. I've come to realise that life is lived moment by moment.

I read once that most people are never fully present in the here and now because unconsciously they believe that the next moment must be more important than this one, but if we do this then we miss our whole life, which is always in the here and now.

I believe that insurance is paid in good faith for those difficult, unexpected events in our lives and yet I have no control over the actions of the income protection insurer. I comply with their requirements, and I continue to rebuild an income stream within my constraints, yet I feel the weight of expectation on me. Given the way I was treated for the first nine months of my claim, I find it distressing when impromptu assessments or case conferences with my doctor are booked.

For this moment

Some of my chronic health challenges persist. However, my well-being has improved over time and this has made writing this book possible.

I had to reconcile the immense grief and loss I felt at no longer being the trusted advisor and respected consultant with a gift for lateral thinking, trouble-shooting and problem solving. I work differently now, and I am at peace with that. For example, I mind-mapped the chapters then dictated this book using speech-to-text over the course of a year.

Even though at times it has been painful and frustrating, this journey has me back in touch with who I really am and how I want to show up. My granddaughters' have taught me so much about the value of being curious, playful and in the moment and I'm grateful I have the opportunity to make a difference.

It is for these reasons that I share this roadmap to well-being, so that you too can feel empowered while navigating your own chronic health challenges. Take one step at a time. This is a journey, not a race. Join me and let's live the fab life together.

Begin with the end in mind

The energy between you and the external world is in a constant feedback loop. When you 'live' the feeling you seek, you tune your energy to resonate with the material pieces that match. Imagine it, feel it now and live it.
Jarl Forsman and Steve Sekhon

Overview

I'm sharing this information because if you are struggling, as I was, I know how important it is for you to paint a new picture of your future. The picture that you have right now is probably not working for you, so what have you got to lose?

This is also about taking back your personal power. When you've been sick for a long time you've probably seen a lot of specialists, doctors and practitioners. This can feel incredibly disempowering as you only receive information on a need-to-know basis or decisions may be made that you don't understand.

What you'll find in this chapter are three keys for creating your vision, as well as actions to help you get clear on where you're going and why.

To get the most out of this chapter, take some time out for yourself to reflect on the changes that you need within your body, mind and soul.

Get clear in your own mind - what do you need, don't focus on what others want for you.

You may have tried many things, some of which might have worked to some degree. But no doubt you've lost momentum when they didn't sustain your well-being easily or made you feel deprived. You may feel stuck and in a place where you perceive it's difficult for you to take steps forward in your well-being. You may be locked in to your current state, where you feel hopeless because you've been given a label that is unhelpful to your progress.

Even well-meaning family members and friends have their points of view that can keep us stuck or locked in. Maybe in the past others have determined your next step and now you're ready to give yourself the opportunity to feel that you're in charge of your own life-affirming decisions.

It's important to feel anchored to your future while being in the present. Visualising a future that builds hope deep inside will help you create the space to thrive, not merely survive.

Change approach

When we need to change the direction of our well-being, our starting point is with our patterns, mindset and behaviours. It's important to follow a process and a framework that helps us to reframe ideas, create new stories and let go of our limiting beliefs.

Here is an approach to change that I work with in my coaching practice and in this book.

The first step is to have a clear REASON for the change. Why is this important to you? Why now?

The second step is a powerful DESIRE. What is the purpose of this change? What will the benefits be for you, not only now but for the long term?

The third step is a COMMITMENT. What is your commitment to action that builds momentum over time, rather than doing what is convenient right now?

These first three steps will support you to explore and validate what you need in order to move forward. Once you have these, they enable you to visualise a future.

The fourth step is a WAY. How will you bring your REASON, DESIRE and COMMITMENT into being? What small actionable steps can you take today, next week, next month?

The fifth step is to find the right level of SUPPORT. What type and level of support do you need to take your small actionable steps? We need shoulder-to-shoulder support, and that's where the work of holistic well-being coaches is vital to so many.

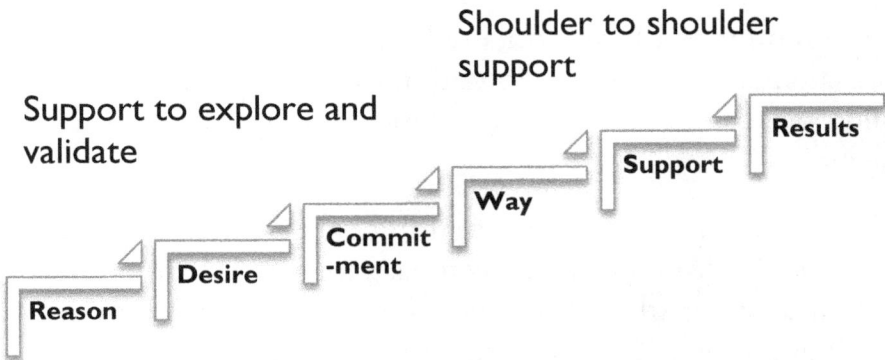

Shoulder to shoulder support

Support to explore and validate

Results

Support

Way

Commit -ment

Desire

Reason

In my view, there are three elements of SUPPORT we can't be without:

- Firm loving kindness that helps us be accountable for doing what we say we will do,
- The space to be honest about our struggles and not feel judged, and
- The advocacy of someone who can be our spokesperson and cheerleader, who reminds us of our progress thus far.

These steps will create lasting change and RESULTS.

To keep moving forward, we need consistent, not perfect, action. We are human beings so are fallible, however, inaction keeps us stuck.

Your Intention

An Intention is a future-oriented positive and descriptive set of statements. We use an Intention to harness the neuroplasticity of the brain to support our journey to well-being.

Now the brain does not distinguish between fact and fiction and doesn't distinguish between past, present and future. Medal-winning athletes use this property of visualisation to profound effect. The rehearsal in their mind of an event or race has almost as much impact on their performance as if the practise were actually happening to the brain and body.

Take some time now to set and write down your Intention, which covers your REASON, DESIRE and COMMITMENT, in a way that allows you to really connect with all the things you'd love to do, have, be and feel.

Here are a few examples from my life so you get the idea.

Example 1

My reason for desiring well-being is to create a life that's joyful, filled with opportunity and pleasure.

My desire is to actively participate in my granddaughters' lives **so that** they flourish and truly experience the love I have for them.

My Intention is to <u>have</u> more energy to <u>do</u> what I choose to do and when. I will <u>be</u> playful, curious and spontaneous. I will therefore <u>feel</u> more joyful and happy, with a deeper connection to people in my life.

Example 2

My reason for desiring well-being is so that I can make a difference in the world by being exactly who I am.

My desire is to create an online show, with interviews that build new insights into holistic well-being, so that people are encouraged to make their health and well-being a priority.

My Intention is to <u>have</u> more clarity and focus, so that I can create and think in alignment with my integrity. I will <u>be</u> happy and content in the knowledge that I am making a difference every day by <u>doing</u> what I love. This helps me <u>feel</u> alive, in touch with my emotions and able to express myself healthfully and with grace.

Once you have crafted your Intention, make it visible. This could include creating a graphic to use as a screensaver on your computer or phone, or pasting photos of your Intention on your mirror, your refrigerator, or in fact, anywhere you will see it frequently.

Once you have created it, read it out loud as often as you can. It is especially powerful when you do this in front of the mirror. Feel into the emotion of that future to embody it. Really practise what it will feel like to 'live as if' it has already happened.

For help with this activity, head to www.hopeinadarktunnel.com to download your free guidebook.

Your future yardstick

When I use traditional success measures - you know the ones I mean... the smart goals: specific, measurable, achievable, realistic and time-bound — what I have found is that I start using what I call my driving energy.

What I mean by driving energy is a pure focus on the goal, and attainment of the goal, rather than focusing on my journey to the outcome with ease and grace.

You really do need alternative measures when looking at your future health and well-being when you are coming from a place of being significantly ill.

This is where your Intention is going to be key, because your success measures will be more around how you feel, how you will be, what you will have and what you will do with that new sense of well-being.

I encourage you to make your future yardstick or benchmark based on improvement from the day that you were at your sickest.

Comparing ourselves to who we were before we became ill is not helpful. It creates a greater sense of hopelessness than anything else I've experienced, because there is often grief attached to the loss of who you thought you were.

An alternative is to use your values. When you understand what you value in your life, you will be able to put your attention, intention and focus to move yourself towards that outcome with ease.

Understanding what you value will support you to choose the most appropriate way of working towards the actions you take.

See the chapter sub-section, *A guiding framework*, for more detail on values.

Take action

- Set and write down your Intention, which covers your REASON, DESIRE and COMMITMENT.
- Make your Intention visible and read it aloud as often as you can.
- Set and write down your success measures.

Wrestling with feeling ill

It's more important to understand the imbalances in your body's basic systems and restore balance, rather than name the dis-ease and match the pill to the ill.
Mark Hyman, MD

Overview

I'm sharing this information because it's key to explore why we feel the need to name what is ailing us before we act.

I don't strictly subscribe to the views that 'we brought things on ourselves', 'we need to learn a lesson' or the woo-woo version 'we manifested it'. However, there are likely choices that we've made that are less-than-optimal for our well-being.

Our aim is to find acceptance in the understanding that we have each made choices and there are consequences to those choices. The key moving forward is to find acceptance where we are right now.

What you'll find in this chapter is food for thought about your past conditioning around health and well-being and some practical techniques to reach acceptance.

I found that I was wrestling with feeling ill because I had a lifetime of 'soldiering on' and prided myself in not taking time off when I was sick. It was difficult to accept that I was so ill and had not paid attention to the signals my body had been giving me.

To get the most out of this chapter you need to be willing to take ownership of your current situation and open yourself to the opportunity of forgiving yourself and others.

Naming the beast

With Western medicine, we have been conditioned to believe that we need a name for what is causing us to feel out of balance. This process of naming or labelling can create a bigger frustration, that of not knowing what's wrong or how to treat an unnamed dis-ease.

If I had stayed stuck in that space, waiting for years for a name or label when the doctors had no answers for me, I would not be at the place in my well-being journey that I am now.

If you look at the 'name it, blame it and give it a pill' method, you quickly find that it is limiting and often exacerbates the problem by putting our focus on the symptoms, not the cause.

The following is an example that illustrates this.

If you are experiencing indigestion (named acid reflux), the western trained doctor will likely ask you about the symptoms you're experiencing. They would probably rule out a hiatus hernia then prescribe you a pharmaceutical drug to reduce the pH of the stomach acid.

These pharmaceutical medications disrupt what the stomach was intended to do. It's an acidic environment designed to break down our food to make it digestible, the nutrients absorbable, as well as protect us from pathogens.

As an aside, a teaspoon of bicarbonate of soda or apple cider vinegar in a little water would provide temporary relief too, but I digress.

What I believe we need most is to look at the problem holistically to find the root cause(s).

In this example we would explore:

- What's your stress level like? What are you doing to manage that?
- Have you recently experienced strong emotions? How have you healthfully expressed these?
- What is your level of exercise each day? Do you get outdoors daily?
- Do you notice what type of foods improve or create more of the problem with indigestion?
- Has your diet changed? What are you doing to maintain a healthy weight?
- How are you eating your meals? When are you eating?

If we pay attention to the signals our body is giving us we could look at each of the four aspects - physical, mental, emotional, soulful - to see where we are out of balance. The following questions help tease this information out:

What difference will it make to you if you have a name or a label?

Would it be wise to explore what your body is telling you and find the root cause(s) of your symptom(s)?

Would it be wise to get the foundations of eating real food, moving more and sleeping well, in place?

Would it be wise to explore and ensure all four aspects of your body are in balance?

Once we understand the root cause(s) we are better equipped to work on a holistic plan to move forward in our well-being.

At one point I was given a name for the chronic health challenges I was experiencing. The name or label of chronic fatigue syndrome (CFS) is a collection of some of the symptoms that I have experienced.

Did it define me? No. Did it help me? Certainly not.

A name or label can be incredibly limiting because you get lumped into a certain category of treatments or perspectives that someone holds. It may mean that you stop paying attention to the body's signals.

You may also take on limiting beliefs, like it not being possible to get well again. For me, a notable example of overcoming this comes from Dr Ian Gawler, who conquered cancer. You can find a link to the article describing his history and experiences in *Section 4 - Wrestling with feeling ill* of the Resources chapter at the end of this book.

You are unique, and your body experiences the highs and lows of life uniquely, so there is seldom a one-size-fits-all approach.

Taming the beast

You will likely have your own beast taming experience and that is why I have shared my journey with you, so you know you are not alone.

When I shared that I was recovering from chronic fatigue syndrome (CFS), I had well-meaning friends and family tell me to exercise more and that would improve my energy. Or they'd ask the timeless and sometimes valid question, "Was I depressed?" The worst experience by far though was people not believing me because apparently, I looked so well.

There is no concrete testing for CFS and the best the medical system has to offer are factors that are found to be present in *most* people.

When you don't fit a label or a definition you can be treated dismissively, which is a rather painful experience.

Reaching acceptance

Step 1

The first step to reaching acceptance, I believe, is understanding the need to let go of

- feeling you're a victim,
- being in the mindset where the situation is hopeless, and
- the feeling that you're helpless.

The limitation of playing the role of the victim is that we stay stuck where we are. I don't perceive an upside to well-being when playing the victim role.

Yes, we may have unknowingly or knowingly contributed to our chronic health challenge. Yes, we may have life events that accelerated our chronic health challenge. Yes, we may have external factors that have contributed to our chronic health challenge. However, if we maintain a victim mindset around our well-being, we can only stay where we are right now. If the status quo is not your preferred option, then what is your possibility?

Step 2

The second step is to decide to take ownership from this moment forward.

Can you choose to let go of feeling hard done by?

Can you choose to let go of feeling that your body has failed you in some way?

Can you choose to let go of feeling that you don't deserve this?

Can you choose to let go of the 'should haves', 'what ifs' and 'if onlys'?

Each choice and each decision we have consciously or unconsciously made has brought us to this place. And we have the power to choose, every day, to move towards what we need instead of staying stuck in this place of limbo.

Step 3

The third step is to forgive yourself and others.

Forgiveness is a powerful forward motivator. Holding onto anger, hurt, abandonment, fear or resentment does nothing to change the past. However, these feelings will affect your future if you indulge in them. Forgiveness is not about condoning or ignoring what has happened but rather about your own healing and wholeness. Petrea King, CEO of Quest for Life Foundation says: "Forgiveness is the foundation of healing", and I agree.

There are autoimmune and other dis-eases that can be linked back to unresolved emotional trauma in your life, so this may be part of the journey you are on. The research article in *Section 4 - Wrestling with feeling ill* of the Resources chapter may prove helpful in these circumstances.

If you do identify with this, you may require professional help to resolve your situation. Seeking the specific help that's needed at an appropriate time is all a part of taking ownership of your situation.

Letting go

What follows is an uncomplicated way to let go, with forgiveness, so that you can move forward. You may have a spiritual practice that you are already comfortable with, so you may choose that to help you release what's not serving you.

Step 1

It will be helpful to reflect and identify the thoughts that come to mind around how you got to this place of being so ill. Note the feeling that you attach to it. If it feels emotionally charged in some way, you need to address it.

Step 2

Write a list of the things that you feel you need to forgive yourself for.

For example, you may have been making poor choices about food because you believed that you were too busy to stop, plan and prepare nourishing food to fuel your body. Or, like me, you did not prioritise managing your stress.

Step 3

Once you have a self-forgiveness list you then write a list of the things to forgive others for.

For example, you may have been exposed to toxic chemicals that have impacted your immune system. Or an important relationship may have disintegrated. Write all these things down.

Step 4

It is then really empowering to use an effective healing practice such as Ho'oponopono, an ancient Hawaiian modality.

The four elements of Ho'oponopono are:

1. Apology - I'm sorry
2. Forgiveness - Please forgive me
3. Gratitude - Thank you
4. Love - I love you

Here is an example of how you can use this practice either silently or out loud:

1. I acknowledge the part I played in (the issue) in my life and I'm sorry.
2. Please forgive me.
   (Repeat this sincerely several times as you recall your apology in #1.)
3. Thank you.
   (Thank your body for all it does for you, yourself for being the best you can be, your spiritual leader, your awareness etc.)

4. I love you.
   (Say it to your body, to your chronic health
   challenges, the air you breathe, the food that
   nourishes you, the house that shelters you, your
   family and friends.)

Do this practice often until the emotional charge of your
feelings is no longer there. You would then follow the same
process for forgiving others, naming and forgiving each in
turn.

Take action

- Pay attention to the signals your body is giving you.
  Look at each of the four aspects - physical, mental,
  emotional, soulful - to see where one is out of
  balance.
- Complete the reaching acceptance activity.
- Complete the letting go activity.

Explore the road to here

Dealing with physical, emotional and psychological issues is much easier if we have a regular practice of looking within, acknowledging and trying to understand our role in every experience.
Jarl Forsman and Steve Sekhon

Overview

I'm sharing this information because it's important to explore your journey to becoming ill or to dis-ease, so you can take the lessons, let go of what no longer serves you and move forward.

It's my belief that our body is like a house with four rooms, we have four aspects to ourselves that make us whole. These aspects are mental, physical, emotional and soulful.

When one is out of balance it impacts the others.

Often our body has given us signals that we haven't paid attention to and it eventually stops us in our tracks. This is my story.

What you'll find in this chapter is an exploration of two challenges that we face when we build our understanding of what we need to leave behind - the proverbial baggage we carry with us.

The first challenge is being able to honestly appraise this baggage. Over the years you've probably collected a lot of undesirable baggage - heartache, loss, disappointment, jealousy, along with your desirable baggage - joy, excitement, contentment, peace.

The second challenge involves unpacking this baggage and deciding what to repack and take with you on your well-being journey.

Getting the most out of this chapter will involve doing some self-exploration. It will help you understand what contributes to the chronic health challenges that you're facing using a tested technique. This will enable you to prioritise aspects and then work on how you can let go of the baggage that no longer supports you.

Holistic perspective

We will use a holistic perspective when we explore how we got to where we are today and it's important to understand these four aspects of ourselves on our journey.

Many people refer to a concept of body, mind and spirit or body, mind and soul, so a key difference here is that we're expanding this and exploring our journey from the aspects of mental, physical, emotional and soulful.

To illustrate this, consider experiencing a physical symptom. We have a way of perceiving the signals that our body is giving us through past experience or knowledge, and then we ascribe it meaning.

For example, we have a headache. The body is signalling to us that something is not right; we may interpret the sensation as nothing to be concerned about, it's simply a headache.

If you have been of the mindset that each symptom your body gives you requires a pill, then you will likely take some paracetamol or codeine to get rid of your headache.

However, if you look at the body's signals in an all-encompassing way, you could ask questions like

- Mental: What 'stinky' thinking is happening for me? Am I experiencing a stress response?
- Physical: Have I drunk sufficient water? Was this headache triggered by something I ate or drank?
- Emotional: What strong emotions am I feeling? Am I fearful of something?
- Soulful: Where am I experiencing a misalignment of my values? Am I feeling isolated?

After checking in with yourself you would then consider alternative approaches instead of taking a pill.

To illustrate this, here are some ways you could go about this to move forward.

Given the brain is made up of around seventy-five percent water and needs to be hydrated to function well, you'd choose to drink some water first.

Next, you might use a practice such as the Emotional Freedom Technique (EFT), which allows you to release the emotion, to process what's going on for you by talking it out and tapping on it. This works at a physiological (physical bodily function) and psychological (mental and emotional) level and will most likely clear the headache in a few rounds.

See Brad Yates' YouTube channel for examples of EFT in practise. The link is in *Section 5 - Explore the road to here* of the Resources.

You may experience tight muscles in your neck from stress, so laying down on a heat pack while doing some slow belly-breathing could relieve the tension, and likely the headache.

Or, you may simply be exhausted and need a twenty-minute power nap.

Do a mental check of what you ate or drank in the last twenty-four plus hours that was different. You may be reacting to preservatives or known allergens. This insight may require a whole course of action of its own.

If the headache returns persistently, it would be wise to see a practitioner to help you unravel the clues and ensure it is nothing sinister.

A different type of Stocktake

What we're going to do now is to explore these aspects of our body through the lens of life events:

- Sit in a quiet place and contemplate the last seven to fourteen years and record what 'major' life events have occurred.
- Once you have noted these life events, consider what feelings you hold about each event.
- As you think about an event, does it bring up desirable or undesirable feelings? For example, does the memory bring up joy, happiness, pleasure, or sadness, pain, loss?
- If you are short on words to describe the emotion you feel, download a list of emotions to support you to express the appropriate one(s). Examples can be found in *Section 5 - Explore the road to here* of the Resources chapter.
- Record what still holds an emotional charge for you and where this shows up in your body.

We can use this understanding to review the emotional energy centres in our body and how this connects with the chronic health challenges we are experiencing right now.

For example, you may feel an intense sense of loss and sadness about the demise of a relationship and when you think about it you experience a tightening of your throat. For me, a major life event where I experienced feelings of rejection and sadness, aligned with the onset of life threatening heart palpitations.

The following diagram shows where in our bodies certain emotional stressors show up and may assist you in completing this activity. It's an unusual way of taking stock of your road to here, however it will help you to understand the integrative nature and connection between the mental, physical, emotional and soulful aspects of yourself.

Once you've joined the dots between your life events, emotions and chronic health challenges, you may need time to process this.

Emotional energy centres

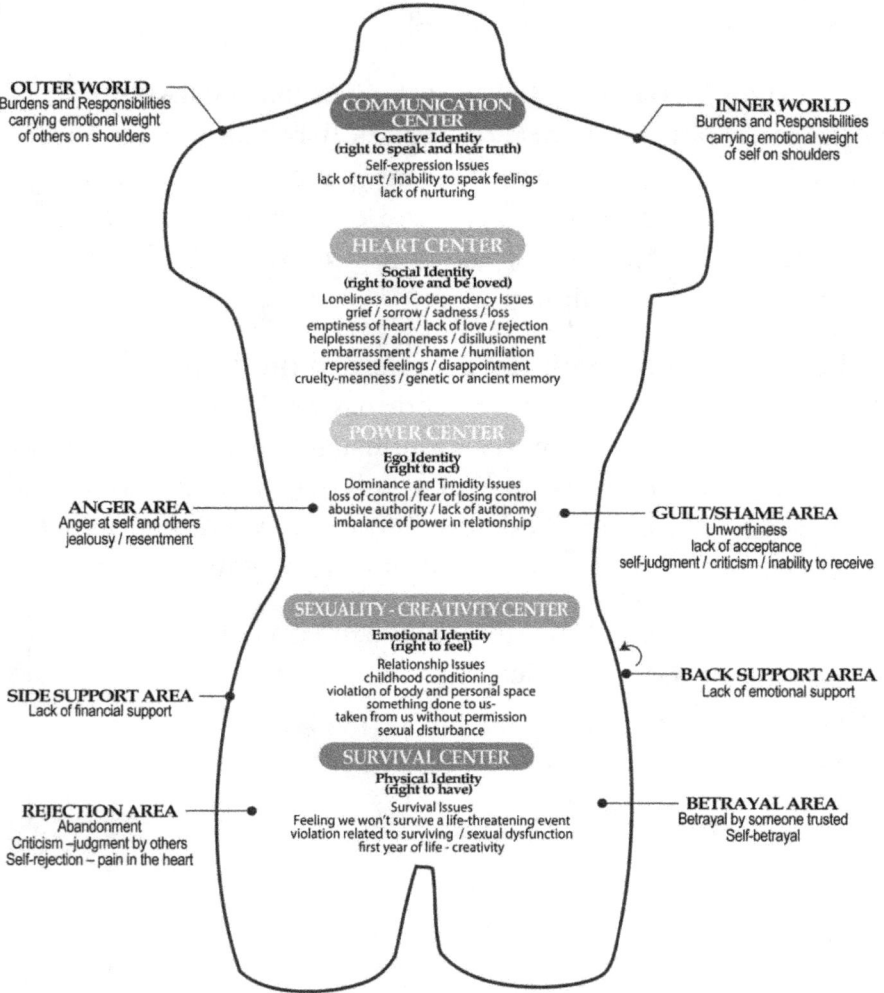

OUTER WORLD
Burdens and Responsibilities
carrying emotional weight
of others on shoulders

INNER WORLD
Burdens and Responsibilities
carrying emotional weight
of self on shoulders

COMMUNICATION
CENTER
Creative Identity
(right to speak and hear truth)
Self-expression Issues
lack of trust / inability to speak feelings
lack of nurturing

HEART CENTER
Social Identity
(right to love and be loved)
Loneliness and Codependency Issues
grief / sorrow / sadness / loss
emptiness of heart / lack of love / rejection
helplessness / aloneness / disillusionment
embarrassment / shame / humiliation
repressed feelings / disappointment
cruelty-meanness / genetic or ancient memory

POWER CENTER
Ego Identity
(right to act)
Dominance and Timidity Issues
loss of control / fear of losing control
abusive authority / lack of autonomy
imbalance of power in relationship

ANGER AREA
Anger at self and others
jealousy / resentment

GUILT/SHAME AREA
Unworthiness
lack of acceptance
self-judgment / criticism / inability to receive

SEXUALITY - CREATIVITY CENTER
Emotional Identity
(right to feel)
Relationship Issues
childhood conditioning
violation of body and personal space
something done to us-
taken from us without permission
sexual disturbance

SIDE SUPPORT AREA
Lack of financial support

BACK SUPPORT AREA
Lack of emotional support

SURVIVAL CENTER
Physical Identity
(right to have)
Survival Issues
Feeling we won't survive a life-threatening event
violation related to surviving / sexual dysfunction
first year of life - creativity

REJECTION AREA
Abandonment
Criticism –judgment by others
Self-rejection – pain in the heart

BETRAYAL AREA
Betrayal by someone trusted
Self-betrayal

Image Credit: Balanced Women's Blog

Reality check

Having completed our Stocktake, we have more information to work from as we explore our journey to here. Now we need to discern what impacts our health and well-being that is within or out of our control. It is here that we explore your role and the role of your physical environment. In the next chapter we will talk about your doctor's role.

Your role

What follows is my Integrative Aspects Model (I.AM) for enquiry. I developed this to act as a compass, so we can check-in with ourselves holistically.

Reflect on the following statements from each aspect of your body. You will get the best results when you can do this truthfully, with a sense of curiosity and without judgement.

I.AM Enquiry

MENTAL ASPECT	SOULFUL ASPECT
I am cultivating 'fragrant' thoughts and self-talk	I am clear on the purpose for my life at this time
I am taking responsibility for my behaviours and actions	I am living aligned with my values each day
I am open to new perspectives or different opinions	I am connecting with people who are uplifting
PHYSICAL ASPECT	**EMOTIONAL ASPECT**
I am making daily choices to deeply nourish my body	I am bouncing back from setbacks with ease
I am valuing daily activity and movement	I am feeling my emotions fully and don't suppress or label them
I am prioritising rest and quality sleep each day	I am expressing my emotions healthfully, with care for myself and others

© Living Fabulously

Wherever you have answered NO, sit with this in contemplation, without judgement, and then journal by hand what comes to mind.

Some helpful questions are:

- How has this way of being kept me safe thus far?
- What's the problem and why do I need to do anything at all?
- What do I need to change and why?
- What are my feasible options and their pros / cons?
- What is the best option for me based on either experience, intuition or what I am willing to give a go right now?
- How will I achieve this change? What actions do I need to take and when will I implement these?
- What obstacles may I face?
- What support do I need to stay on track?

For help with this activity head to www.hopeinadarktunnel.com to download your free guidebook.

If there is an area where you feel you are struggling, then be courageous and seek the right level of support for yourself. Remember, you have the opportunity to make choices that are right for you.

Role of the physical environment

With the advent of the industrial age, the environment has changed dramatically from that of our ancestors. This modernisation has not been without a price on our health and well-being.

It's critical for you to consider the ways that you're interacting with your physical environment, as it is a key contributor to your current state of health.

In simple terms, when you remove the stressors in your physical environment, your immune system has more opportunity to do its vital work.

When I say physical environment, I am including

- noise levels,
- quality of air,
- quality of food, and
- chemicals in household and personal products.

This topic could be a whole book in itself, so if you need to know more, examine the information and reliable websites in *Section 5 - Explore the road to here* of the Resources chapter.

Noise and Air Quality

Noise exposure can have a negative influence on your well-being by increasing your level of stress, which in turn can lead to a raised heart rate and unhealthy blood pressure.

I left a busy city because the air pollution, traffic noise and busyness of the city jangled my nerves terribly and worsened my symptoms. A small, quiet beachside suburb was much more appropriate for me and it's where I've made the most leaps forward in my well-being journey. The suburb I live in is surrounded by National Park / Forest, which means the oxygen is high and air pollution low.

Oxygen is pivotal to the functioning of your immune system. But what if you do live in the city? You can buy an air purifier or use a Himalayan Salt Lamp to compensate to some degree however on weekends it would be important to spend time in nature, even if it's just sitting on a bench in a park.

For me, the beach is within walking distance, so I regularly get my dose of negative ions, with the added benefit of feeling grounded by being in nature.

Moving water (think mountain streams, waterfalls and beaches) has the unique property of creating elevated levels of negative ions. Studies have shown that negative ions increase levels of your 'happy hormone' (serotonin), helping to lift your mood, relieve stress and stimulate your energy. So, getting a dose of these ions whenever you can will help improve your well-being.

What if you don't live near moving water? You can buy negative ion generators, which are a reasonable substitute. I bought one that was a small 'tower' shape and ran it in my apartment while I lived in the city, and I still use this in my office now. I experienced an increased sense of well-being and relaxation especially knowing that the air was cleared of dust, pollen and mould spores.

Food Quality

Our food is not what it was in previous generations. The soil has been depleted of its minerals and nutrients through the advent of monoculture. In big-business agriculture, crops are no longer rotated, and fields are never allowed to lie fallow to rest and regenerate. And with mechanisation came crop spraying using toxic chemicals, e.g. glyphosate.

Glyphosate is commonly called Round Up all over the world. A potent weed killer, it is also a neurotoxin that has devastating impacts on the human body and has been attributed to the rise of autoimmune illnesses and other inflammatory dis-eases. Relevant research articles can be found in *Section 5 - Explore the road to here* of the Resources chapter.

Therefore, eating organic and locally grown food is a critical step on your well-being journey. Fresh organic whole foods are needed to derive the most nutritional value, as these have loads of micronutrients that can support your healing.

I am fortunate to have access to a local farmers market where I can buy organic and chemical-free fresh produce every Sunday morning. But what if you don't have access to organically grown food?

Then educating yourself on the 'dirty dozen' and 'clean fifteen' lists of fresh produce (See links in Section 5 - Explore the road to here of the Resources chapter) is even more important. The 'dirty dozen' are a list of foods with pesticide residue that must be avoided unless organic. The 'clean fifteen' are a guide if you can't source organic foods.

Be sure to rinse your fresh produce in lightly salted water (made with Celtic sea salt or Himalayan salt) to clean off any surface residue, especially any non-organic produce.

Become an avid label reader if you must resort to buying food products in a bag, box or can. Just because a food product in a bag, box or can is labelled organic, that doesn't necessarily mean it is healthy for you. If you see numbers and names you can't pronounce, put the food-like substance back on the shelf.

Chemical Exposure

Our skin is the largest organ of the body and what we apply to it is absorbed into our bloodstream. If it is toxic, it quickly becomes a burden on an already overworked immune system.

In addition, when we use household products we inhale the vapours, and these have a direct impact on our health. Be mindful of the ingredients in topical products as well as household products. And, be aware that there can be declared or undeclared concoctions of hazardous chemicals that act as endocrine system disruptors, have carcinogenic properties and act as neurotoxins in the body.

I strongly recommend referring to the *Starter list of* Toxic Chemicals in *Section 5 - Explore the road to here* of the Resources chapter for more information.

The investment in organic products is a pro-active and preventative step toward relieving the toxic burden on your immune system.

The cost of organic products in the short term will future-proof your health in the long term. Think of the investment as health insurance to avoid the risk of dis-ease. Your body will thank you.

Take action

- Complete your Stocktake activity.
- Make time to reflect on what your Stocktake has revealed.
- Respond to the questions in the I.AM Enquiry model.
- Sit in contemplation with your NO answers and then journal by hand what comes to mind.
- Note what needs to change in your physical environment short, medium and long term.

Experience of normalising the abnormal

Only we can decide what will work best to make us feel good.
We are the navigators and adventurers on our
totally unique journey.
Jarl Forsman and Steve Sekhon

Overview

I'm sharing this information because time plays tricks on us. When we are ill, over time, we create a new normal. We lose sight of what true health and well-being are for us.

Over time we come to accept, for example, that results on a blood test are our normal, yet if you compared them to a few years before, or even sometimes a few months before, they would not be our normal.

What often results is that because of this new normal, the doctor may find your blood results acceptable. Therefore, your treatment plan begins to ignore the fact that you still hadn't uncovered the root cause(s).

This happened to me. I had an unusual white blood cell count and it was listed on my blood results as mild neutropenia. After two years of seeing that same result, my doctor at the time declared that my blood results were normal. However, I had never had mild neutropenia reported on any blood results prior to this time. I discussed this with the doctor because I recognised this was not my normal. I now know it indicated the underlying chronic infection that had gone untreated for many years.

What we will explore in this chapter is a perspective on what true health and well-being means for you. You need to understand and discern the signals that your body gives, listen carefully and take appropriate action. What's implicit here is understanding your role in your health, versus your practitioner's role.

The way you will do this is by taking a big picture audit of your health and well-being. This will help you distinguish between the cause and effect, so you will be better equipped for the part you play in your well-being journey.

What good health and well-being looks like

I believe that good health and well-being is not merely the absence of dis-ease. We often create a new normal about the state of our health and well-being, and then accept that this is how things will be.

The boiling frog parable describes a frog being slowly boiled alive. So, it is with declining health.

If a frog is put suddenly into boiling water, it will jump out. So, if we were suddenly faced with a health crisis, we'd take immediate action. For example, if you tripped and fell, breaking your arm, you would hot-foot it to emergency and have it seen to.

However, if the frog is put in tepid water that is then brought to the boil slowly, it will not perceive the danger and will die. The truth is, your body is giving you signs and signals that danger is ahead, however, we often accept things such as joint pain, headaches or digestive upset as our new normal. We become the frog in the second scenario.

To me, good health and well-being mean that I have the freedom to do what I choose to do and how I want to do it. It's the vitality, that real joy and essence of life, that makes me feel good and have the energy to do what I love.

Pause for a moment and reflect on what good health and well-being would look like for you.

Is it that you can do meaningful work and create a source of income?

Is it that you can choose to go for a walk along the beach?

Is it that you have the energy to play with your children or grandchildren?

It may be all the above, and that is why the Intention we created earlier helps us to navigate the change we need for our well-being.

The story you've been telling yourself

How in touch are you with your body and its signals? What symptoms or ailments have you been experiencing that you've chosen to ignore or have perhaps normalised? How have you been adapting your lifestyle to suit your symptoms?

How often are you saying
it's just [fill in the blank, e.g. a headache, joint pain],
so it must be [fill in the blank, e.g. my eyes, old age],
OR, you resort to popping a pill with no exploration?

The body is a highly integrated and well-designed set of systems and processes. Each component of the body has a specific role, or several roles, to play in keeping the physical and mental body in good shape. When we take time to notice that something feels out of balance, we can then take steps to understand the underlying causes.

This is when we can use the I.AM questions (in the *I.AM Enquiry* section from the chapter *Explore the road to here*) to discover where the problem may lie. It is here that we can find out if the symptom stems from a mental, physical, emotional or soulful aspect.

Your role vs your practitioner's role

You play a vital role in your health and well-being journey. You are the one who needs to take control in a way that provides your practitioner with what they need to best support you.

When you arrive at your appointment, the practitioner has usually not had the opportunity to review all your notes to date, so they're relying on you to provide a concise account of what's happened in the past period, how you're responding to the treatment plan and so forth.

It's important to note that the tests that the practitioner has ordered are just one measure of your health at a particular point in time.

To complement the I.AM enquiry and uncover a pattern with recurring or infrequent symptoms, a useful digital tool that works on Android and iPhone smartphones is "*mySymptoms Diary*". Find the link in *Section 6 – Experience of normalising the abnormal* of the Resources chapter.

I use this with my clients as they can record things such as

- stress intensity and duration,
- mood on a scale of 1 to 5, with space for notes,
- symptom intensity and duration,
- energy levels and duration,
- sleep quality and duration,
- exercise intensity and duration,
- food - broken down by meal,
- bowel movement using the Bristol Scale, and
- medications and / or supplements.

The recorded information can be shared as a PDF on email, so becomes a valuable tool in our coaching sessions, as we can then explore this to create insight and promote action.

Using a tool like *mySymptoms* to monitor and measure other factors around your health and well-being also means you provide a much richer canvas for the practitioner to work on with you, rather than simply relying on memory.

You may have test results, which could be inconclusive. However, your broader clinical picture is enormously important in your treatment plan as it adds detail to, and possibly provides explanation for, some of the things you are experiencing. It is made up of your constellation of symptoms, responses to medication or supplements, and the changes (for the better or worse) in the symptoms you've experienced to date, all of which can aid a diagnosis.

When your practitioner gives you suggestions and recommendations to implement, make a note of the actions to take and be sure you understand exactly what they are asking of you. Your role, post the appointment, is to be consistent with your implementation.

Take action

- Reflect on what good health and well-being would look like for you.
- Update your Intention if required.
- Track recurring or infrequent symptoms or other aspects of well-being for at least four weeks.
- Explore the underlying patterns you observe in the data.

Journey through the medical system

*We don't want band-aids for our symptoms. We want to get to
the root cause. We don't want to be treated as a body part —
we want to be understood as a whole person.*
Mark Hyman, MD

Overview

I share this information with you because your appointment
with the practitioner is merely a snapshot in time. It's a
necessity to take back our personal power, especially when it
comes to working with practitioners.

Dr Frank Lipman says: "So until we can rely on Doctors to
teach us prevention or how to maintain health, it is essential
that you the reader gets educated and takes responsibility for
your own health care".

I agree with Dr Frank Lipman that we need to be
responsible for our own health care. When you're on a
journey through the medical system, it is stressful to make
decisions. You feel bombarded with a whole lot of, often
conflicting, information that's made even more challenging
when you're feeling ill. My desire here is to share tools which
you can utilise to minimise that stress.

What you will find in this chapter is how to

- make an informed choice that is right for you,
- find the right practitioner for you,
- summarise and maintain your health history, and
- make effective use of the cost of your practitioner
  visits.

To get the most out of this chapter you will determine what choices are available to you and create your health summary. This health summary ensures that your practitioner has the right information at their fingertips at any point in time.

I understand, and know first-hand, that it can be hard when you are not experiencing change or progress over a longer period. However, we need to learn to trust ourselves and our body's ability to heal, even more than we trust our practitioners.

Our bodies have infinite wisdom and when we get in touch with and tune in to our body's signals, it leads to more healing than if we relied on external inputs alone.

Your choices

I perceive that there are four main branches of medicine that can support you in your well-being journey:

1. Western Medicine,
2. Traditional Medicine,
3. Complementary Medicine, and
4. Functional and Integrative Medicine.

The table that follows aims to illustrate the principles of each of these four branches and highlights the specificity of each one. Errors and omissions are completely mine as this is a vast topic that I have endeavoured to summarise.

	Western Medicine	Traditional Medicine	Complementary Medicine	Functional & Integrative Medicine
Type of practitioner	• General doctors • Specialist doctors • Allied practitioners e.g. physiotherapist	• Traditional Chinese Medicine • Acupuncture • Ayurvedic Medicine • Homeopathic Medicine	• Chiropractic • Osteopathy • Naturopathy • Kinesiology • Hypnotherapy	• Doctors who combine Western Medicine, some evidence-based Traditional and Complementary Medicine with scientific research
Approach	• Diagnosis based on clinical presentation • Treatment of symptoms with pharmaceutical or surgical interventions by Doctors • Treatment with a defined therapy from allied practitioners	• Diagnosis using the whole physical body • Treatment with herbs, tincture, or extracts to stimulate the body's healing systems and create balance	• Diagnosis based on the whole physical body, mind body connection and energetic body • Treatment of emotional, physical and energetic body depending on modality	• Less concerned with making a diagnosis and more concerned with the underlying imbalances • Treating the patient not the dis-ease
Focus	• Suppression of dis-ease • Treat acute situations	• Working from a holistic perspective	• Creating balance and harmony in the body	• Creating a therapeutic partnership toward well-being

Find links to some of the practitioners I follow in *Section 7 - Journey through the medical system* of the Resources chapter.

How to find a Functional or Integrative Medicine Practitioner

Step 1: Understand what you need

- Know what your primary well-being issues are, as functional or integrative medicine doctors may be generalists or specialists.
- Know that there is no single definition of functional medicine.
- There is no single place where doctors can receive training in functional medicine.
- Functional medicine is not always covered by health insurance.
- Just because a doctor is listed on a website or says they do functional medicine, that does not mean they're competent.

Step 2: Do your high-level research

- Ask for a referral from your own network, support group or forum.
- Do a Google search and Google map search for "functional medicine and (town name)" and see what results you get. Do the same for surrounding towns and similar keywords.
- Determine what the reputable credentialed or certified bodies are for your country.

I found some links for members and alumni of institutions (mainly American oriented) and posted these in *Section 7 - Journey through the medical system* of the Resources chapter.

Step 3: In-depth research to create a shortlist

- Explore the practitioner's website(s) and confirm their listed credentials.
- Read their blog(s).
- Find them on Facebook and read the reviews.
- Find them on Google and review articles, especially publications.
- Find them on YouTube and get an experience of them on video.
- If they have a book, read the reviews online, or preferably read the book yourself.

As you are researching, consider the following:

- What level of confidence do you feel having read the information?
- Have they blogged or talked about your specific health challenges?
- Do you feel comfortable with their treatment approach?
- Does it seem as if you will get along well with them?

Step 4: Investigate your shortlist

Contact the practitioner's office. Will they do a free / low cost phone consultation with new patients? Doing this means that you can both be sure you're a good fit before going further. It will let you get to know the doctor and ask a few questions with little to no risk.

I paid for an initial consultation with a functional medicine doctor who seemed to tick my boxes online, yet in person, I lost confidence in his rigid treatment protocol and his manner. However, I did receive confirmation that I was dealing with a chronic infection.

Being an investigator with a trusted partner

Imagine you're commanding officer Olivia Benson from Law & Order: SVU or DB Russell from CSI, and you have a trusted partner(s) who works on the case with you. Two heads are better than one for sure.

When I was extremely ill, I didn't have the capacity to ask the right questions or to retain the information. My strategy to deal with this was to have a good friend or my daughter come to my medical appointments as an impartial observer. This support person was able to prompt me with questions prepared beforehand if I lost my train of thought and to take notes when required.

When major decisions need to be made about your treatment plan, your trusted partner can support you. It may be by synthesising the pros and cons they took notes on, to help you explore what the right choice is for you.

It's possible that your life partner or immediate family member may not be the right person to fill this role, so consider someone who cares about you, is pragmatic and who can be impartial when presenting the options to you.

The type of things you need to ask your practitioner will depend on the type of practitioner you are seeing, the nature of your health challenge and where you are on your well-being journey.

However, here are some helpful guidelines:

- What is the underlying cause of the symptom?
- What is the meaning of the term you used?
- What are the alternatives to... (e.g. treatment / medication / supplements)?

- What are the pros and cons?
- What are the likely side effects?
- What are the interactions with the medication or supplements I am already taking?
- What are the expected outcomes and timeframes?

Create a list of questions you need to ask before you go to your appointment and have this on hand, along with your up to date health summary.

Your health summary

When you've been ill for a long time, your practitioner does not have the time to read through your copious medical records. Whilst they may have recall of who you are and the headline problems, they may not recall all the intricate details. Therefore, having your health summary is vital to making headway with the practitioner and avoiding unnecessary expense.

Each practitioner has a scope of practice and so they know what is within their remit to support you best. In other words, they are "working within their zone of genius", as we say in the business world.

So, the best use of your time and money with your practitioner is to present information in a concise way and to provide them with a summary that highlights the salient points.

I find that maintaining four sections in my health summary ensures the practitioner is up to date quickly and this proves effective.

These four sections are:

1. Medical events and date of occurrence.
2. Chronology of tests and outlier results (i.e. top, bottom or outside the test scale).
3. Current medication and supplements including the brands and dosages.
4. Continuous versus intermittent symptoms, including their intensity, duration and frequency.

For help with this activity, head to www.hopeinadarktunnel.com to download your free guidebook.

Take action

- Complete the activity to find a Functional or Integrative Medicine Practitioner.
- Find a trusted partner who meets your requirements.
- Create your health summary.

Finding your support crew

True friends are concerned about each other's well-being and are naturally inclined to help one another attain it. They provide positive support that is uplifting and life enhancing.
Jarl Forsman and Steve Sekhon

Overview

I share this information with you because sometimes your immediate or nuclear family don't understand where you're at and can't comprehend why you're not getting better quickly. You feel frustrated with the, "Why don't you just [fill in the blank]" advice being dished out.

Your support crew need to provide you with a sounding board, so you can talk things out without judgement and have the opportunity to recognise and solve your own problems. Another important thing is to recognise how people's energy can impact yours and vice versa, so it's about finding the right level of support for you that can lift or maintain your energy at all times.

What you'll find in this chapter are ways to identify and create the right support crew. This chapter will also help you become clear on your needs, so that you know exactly what sort of support you're going to need to move forward. It's also key to understand the history you have with your family and friends, so that you can be sure about what is yours and what is not yours to own and to manage.

To get the most out of this chapter you need to create clarity around your own needs and we will be doing that in a specific activity. Following that, you will have the opportunity to find out what forms of support work best for you.

It can be difficult for some people to put their hand up for support; many of us have been completely independent for many reasons. We need strategies for dealing with unsupportive people and the burdens we feel they place on us, as we're working towards well-being, just as we do in other areas of our lives.

What do you need?

First and foremost, it is not your job to convince anyone that you're ill. A lot of people are well meaning yet may have no understanding of chronic health challenges. Many have never experienced this themselves nor have they cared for someone in such a situation.

It may be that they looked to you for strength or guidance and don't relate to you when you're ill. For example, you may have been the 'strong one' in your family or network and people have never witnessed you showing vulnerability, so they may feel uncomfortable with that change. This is not your problem, it is their story to own and solve.

What is important for you to consider is what you need to feel supported and empowered in the decisions that you make in terms of your own well-being.

Do you need practical help e.g. with meals, transport etc.?

Do you need someone who will be your sounding board?

Do you need someone who can help you to create a list of pros and cons around the decision you're about to make?

Do you need someone to listen to you to express your thoughts, concerns and fears openly?

Do you need unconditional support for your choices - someone who will hear your darkest deepest fears and the unburdening of your heart without trying to fix it?

Do you need someone who has a balanced perspective?

Do they impartially observe the upside or the downside of situations?

Do you trust their judgement around matters of the heart?

Do you need someone who demonstrates positivity and empathy?

What I mean by positivity is not the Pollyanna principle of everything being all right all the time. Rather, during a challenging situation, they will help you to see what's possible and how to move forward from that place.

Take time to reflect now. What will you need from your support crew?

Empathy is an art and a skill

If we're in a fast-flowing river of despair, uncertainty or hopelessness, we don't need people jumping into the river with us to drown alongside us. We also don't need them standing on the side of the river telling us what to do. What we need is for them to extend a branch from the bank, one we can hang onto.

Empathy in action, for me, is creating time to pause and think your challenge through and to work out how to get back to the bank, with or without support. My suggestion is to surround yourself with people who are both positive and empathetic.

On your way to well-being you will need a whole support crew, as no single person can fulfil every need when you're ill. You certainly don't need to create a co-dependent relationship either.

A group of people who have different things to offer has been so helpful on my well-being journey. They would be a delightful bunch of 'misfits' if I put them in a room together, simply because of their diversity.

I am often enlisted to support my client's needs in several aspects of their journey because as a coach, I am impartial, balanced, empathetic and objective, just what you need in a support person.

Where will you find support?

A safe landing space for emotions

We need people in our lives who are good listeners, who pay attention to what is being said and to what is *not* being said. We need people to listen without judgement and not to try to solve our challenges for us.

Sometimes, talking out what's in our heads helps us to make sense of the turmoil that lies within. So long as this is not a circular or ruminating style of conversation, it may be valuable. However, I believe you have access to all you need, including the wisdom to resolve this turmoil, when you create the space for reflection.

Julia Cameron, author of the *The Artist's Way*, talks about Morning Pages as a method of journaling and I find her practice really supports me. The premise is, as soon as you wake up, sit up in bed with your journal and a pen. Recollect the dreams you have had and write them down, along with everything you can think of to be grateful for. Recall all the aspects of your life for which you have gratitude, no matter how small.

Julia Cameron recommends listing ten gratitude's each day, however, start where you are, even if it's only three to begin with. Next, let your pen flow and write whatever needs to come out and land on your page. This is where you get everything out of your system, good, bad or otherwise. Once it's on the page, it no longer needs to compete for space in your head or heart.

The reason that I love this morning practice is that it doesn't stir up emotions or feelings that may need to be explored, right before going to bed. As a sleep maven, it's a tip I share with all my clients.

If you are new to journaling, purchase yourself a notebook that is aesthetically pleasing to you and keep it on your bedside table with a pen. I've got one that's made from hand woven silk fabric, which I find so beautiful to hold and touch. I find that this really enhances my journaling experience. I've had others that have a quote on the front that is uplifting and supportive. Whatever you choose, make sure it's something you'll want to spend time with.

Your Journal is not the same as a Diary. To me, a Diary is a narrative of events that may have some emotions or feelings attached. The practice of journaling on waking allows you greater access to the subconscious mind, so that you are able to journal what's in your heart.

When you review your journaling from time to time, you may observe a theme or pattern emerging. Be curious as you read and committed to taking courageous action. This may be to seek support, have a conversation or to let go of old hurts. In the section *Letting go* of the chapter *Wrestling with feeling ill*, I shared a process that can help here, so you may need to revisit that section if this is your experience.

You can also find out more about the practice of journaling in *Section 8 - Finding your support crew* of the Resources chapter.

Practical help

You may need practical help with daily living, or even support for when you go to the doctor. Find people in your local network who are most likely to make time available to support you. Often, we are not willing to impose on others, yet that's not what our support crew like us to do.

People can't read our minds, and unless we ask, they wouldn't know that we needed their help. They would want us to reach out when we need them.

Our self-sufficiency really can get in the way of reaching out and making the request.

One example of this strategy is enlisting people to help you batch-cook meals, then freezing portions. It means you won't need to cook each day, yet you'll still have nourishing meals on hand. This worked well for me as it doubled as a social activity too.

If you have a slow cooker, pressure cooker and oven casserole dish, you could have stews, soups and baked options in your freezer by the end of one cook-up.

Another example is in the cleaning of your home. If you have the funds you could outsource this. However, if you don't, you may need to work out some strategies and enlist people. I enjoy and feel energised by a neat and clean home and in the early days of my well-being journey, I could either dust or tidy in one room in a day. My daughter lovingly did the 'heavy cleaning' for me once a week and continues to do so after my granddaughters' have visited and created a happy 'mess'.

I did have to let go of the 'clean freak' in me and place more priority on my well-being, but over time as my strength picked up, I was able to do a little more for myself without setting myself back.

Whatever your need is, be willing to step outside your comfort zone to put your hand up, so that people can support you in a way that is enriching for both of you.

Staying social within constraints

When you're facing chronic health challenges it can be isolating, especially when certain social activities that were your norm feel out of reach.

We are social beings so it's important to be in community with others. It's equally important to manage your own energy and know what your own limits are around socialisation.

Is a short phone call something you value and can do?

How do you go having visitors in your own home?

Is it best for one visitor only, or can you cope with a small number of visitors?

Do you have the energy to go out for a specific amount of time with others?

While you're in a challenging space with your health, you may need to enlist someone else that can observe your body's signals and prompt you to conclude social activities when they notice you begin to decline.

Healthy boundaries you own

While it's important at any time, it is paramount to keep good company when you are ill. You need to surround yourself with positive and uplifting people who won't ignore the fact that you're ill yet can create the space to set it aside for now. We need to recognise that well-being is the priority. Having people in our immediate environment who are negative or who have challenges of their own that they're dealing with (or not), is unhelpful.

It's key that you know your own limits for other areas in your life beyond socialising, such as exercising, networking and working. That's not to say we should stay in our comfort zones. However, if you constantly go past your current levels of stamina and endurance, the likely outcome is setbacks in your health and well-being.

"Everything in moderation" takes on a new meaning when some days all you feel you can do is get out of bed.

Being assertive and explicit about your needs is what I've referenced throughout this chapter. However, if you have not done this before it can feel daunting to set boundaries with people, especially those closest to you.

For me, the most important parts about setting personal boundaries in relationship to others come from your values, beliefs about yourself and your ability to change old patterns of behaviour.

My good friend and colleague, Patti Villalobos is an incredible boundaries, mindfulness and resilience coach and she graciously shares her wisdom on setting personal boundaries with us. Sometimes people stumble when setting boundaries because they don't know how or when to balance firmness, empathy, resolve and respect.

Setting boundaries is sometimes about saying "no" loudly and firmly; and sometimes it's about setting a limit and having a conversation. It depends on the context and the relationship.

Here are the steps Patti teaches when setting boundaries.

Know what's important to you

What's most important to you?

If what's most important is setting your boundary regardless of whether the other person agrees or not, then you come through the RESULTS lens. For example, if someone is yelling or cussing at me and I need him or her to stop now, then that's what's most important.

If speaking up and sharing my truth while I set the boundary is most important, then SELF ESTEEM is the lens to use. For example, if I've been letting my friend walk all over me for months, giving a voice to why it is no longer okay may be important to me.

If I am in a trusting (and the word "trust" is key) relationship, then I might need to set the boundary in a way that is collaborative and win-win for both of us. Here is where I'll enter into a conversation about the boundary as I set it. This is the RELATIONSHIP lens. For example, your partner constantly leaves things lying around and keeping a tidy house is important to you, have a conversation about this to set an agreed boundary.

Results lens

For the RESULTS lens, be firm and resolved.

Firm means the other person does not mistake my "no", so there's no room for wishy-washiness here. Resolved means, I don't question my right to set the boundary, I just do it. If the situation allows, I am neutral or polite, and I avoid inflammatory language. I don't need to start a fight with the person yelling or cussing. But I'm not going for polite, instead I am going for a no-nonsense "stop", with body language and tone of voice that says, "We aren't going to have a discussion about this."

Self esteem lens

For the SELF ESTEEM lens, be brave, respectful and brief.

Brave means I speak up and tell the other person how I feel. Respectful means I don't dump my anger or insult the other person. Brief means I don't allow the interaction to get into a long, drawn-out discussion or fight.

I avoid lectures or accusations, and I stick to using "I" statements to explain myself. When I come through the SELF ESTEEM lens, I'm telling myself and the other person that "I matter".

Relationship lens

For the RELATIONSHIP lens, be empathetic, kind and inclusive.

Empathy allows me to hear the other person, but I don't confuse empathy with backing down. Kind allows me to say my words in a way that the other person can hear them. Finally, because this is a trusting relationship, I need to be collaborative and include the other person in the discussion about what the required boundary looks like.

Practise makes skilled

For all lenses, I give myself grace as I learn to set stronger boundaries and trust that, with practise, my boundaries will become "just the way it is" and won't take so much effort and energy. But any energy I do spend on my boundaries is well worth it…because I am worth it.

Where and with whom do you need to set healthy boundaries?

Find out more about Patti Villalobos' work in *Section 8 - Finding your support crew* of the Resources chapter.

Take action

- Respond to the questions to determine what you need from your support crew.
- Start or continue journaling using a practice like Morning Pages.
- Make a list of requests and determine who in your support crew is a good fit.
- Make contact and ask for the support you need.

- Where and with whom do you need to set healthy boundaries?
- Practice holding your healthy boundaries in areas that you feel most equipped.

Your body - your vehicle for life

*The key to success is to intentionally design your environment to
make it easy to do the right thing and create health.*
Mark Hyman, MD

Overview

I share this information with you so that you can create
health and well-being in a way that's appropriate for you.
We'll explore getting out of any stuckness or out of your
comfort zone in three key areas.

You may feel that your body has let you down. The physical
experience of your chronic health challenge is distressing,
and it is a difficult journey at the best of times. However, if
we don't take care of ourselves it is impossible to create the
right conditions for the body to repair and heal itself. We
need to ensure that our bodies are well nourished, moved
more and well rested.

A critical part of this chapter looks at ways of getting back
to basics, creating a new relationship with our body and
reducing inflammation. What you will find here are ideas for
fuelling your body, reducing inflammation and boosting
your immune system. As with any physical structure, the
body needs solid foundations to withstand the environment.

To get the most out of this chapter, be open to the
possibilities of doing different things AND doing things
differently. Use the content to do a holistic check-in, while
still working within your constraints. Know that each of
your choices today shape your future, so let's choose wisely.

Nourish well

To me, nourishing your body well means eating real food filled with enzymes. I'm talking about food that you would buy in the fresh organic produce aisle of a supermarket, or better still, at your local organic farmer's market. This is nature's bounty.

It's not the food-like substances processed or manufactured in a factory and filled with additives, that come in a bag, box, can or jar, that are void of enzymes. I'm talking about food that comes from Mother Earth, that our bodies know how to digest and use to create energy and vitality.

Our bodies recognise real food and know how to turn this into fuel. The root cause of much dis-ease is linked to inflammation in the body. Eating real, organic, whole foods is a non-inflammatory way of providing your body with nourishment.

The exception may be food intolerances e.g. gluten and dairy. You, like myself, may be sensitive to the deadly nightshade family, which causes inflammation in some. This includes tomatoes, tomatillos, eggplant, white potatoes, goji berries and peppers of all types, including chilli. However, pause for a moment and think of how many other vegetables and fruits there are to choose from.

Many people use the phrase "clean eating", and I love it because it explains that we are eating a colourful rainbow of organic whole foods. When we eat a variety of organic whole foods we are providing our body with the vital macro and micro-nutrients required to build a healthy body.

Crowding out

When you decide to change what you eat and drink, you need to be successful and stick with your choices, as this will motivate you to keep moving forward. One of the keys to success is to crowd out the foods you need to let go of. This will minimise resistance from the brain, and the body adapts as you make small step-by-step changes.

The best way to start with a change in what you eat is to introduce more real, organic food and not pay too much attention to the 'problem' foods immediately.

Crowding out is a concept that allows you to move towards what it is you need, without creating restriction, deprivation or putting focus on the foods that you are letting go of. For example, you may currently be eating a dinner that is mainly meat, has one token vegetable, white potatoes and gravy. The way you would crowd out is to increase the variety of vegetables, so that they cover seventy-five percent of your plate, and add a palm sized serving of protein. Your next steps may be to review what protein sources are more suitable for you, substitute sweet potatoes for the starchy white ones and make a jus, instead of the gravy made with flour.

Say you enjoy eating a lot of pasta, which is a shelf-food that is refined and processed. You could keep the dish the same, except crowd out the pasta by replacing it with organic brown rice or an organic gluten-free ancient grain that's been properly prepared e.g. quinoa. Your next steps may be to consider changes to the sauce or to substitute spiralised zucchini instead of rice or ancient grains.

The last example is the story of a client of mine who drank several sugar-free caffeinated soft drinks a day. She crowded out these drinks by upping the amount of water she was drinking instead. The benefits included no longer feeling tired but wired, improved sleep, and waking up feeling refreshed and energised.

Hydration

Did you know that your body is made up of between sixty to seventy-five percent water? It's no surprise that how much water you drink can affect your health and concentration. Too much water could result in mineral imbalances, while too little could cause dehydration, headaches, or fatigue. Being well hydrated gives your brain and body the boost it needs to function well all day. It's important to realise that beverages such as tea, coffee or soft drinks are dehydrating to the body. Even though they have water added to them, they do not replace the need for pure water.

To calculate how much water to drink you need to factor in how active you are, the heat and your body weight.

Two calculations to approximate your daily water intake are

1. Imperial system (pounds and ounces) - divide your body weight in half and the value is your daily water intake in ounces.
   e.g. Weight = 160 lbs therefore water intake = 80 ounces

2. Metric system (kilograms and litres) - multiply your weight by 0.03 to get your daily water intake in litres
   e.g. Weight = 73 kgs. therefore water intake = 2.2 litres

Aim to drink the purest water you can to minimise the intake of toxins. The best option is a reverse osmosis water filter fitted to your sink, so you have filtered water on tap for drinking and cooking.

A tip to get started is to fill a reasonably sized glass jug or bottle with filtered water and place on your desk or kitchen counter, with the aim being to drink most of it before midday. Often, we mistake thirst for hunger so before you reach for a snack between meals, drink a glass of filtered water.

Many people who have chronic health challenges are highly likely to have digestive issues. Here are my 'liquid' tips to improve digestion:

1. Drink a glass of filtered water or a cup of chamomile tea at least fifteen minutes before a meal.
2. Don't drink water or beverages with your meal.
3. Wait one and a half to two hours after your meal to drink fluids again.

This provides the right conditions for the enzymes and acid in your stomach to properly digest the food.

Inflammatory Foods

With our modern living we have created a situation where we are sensitised to gluten (found in grains), refined sugar and dairy products. Our gut health is compromised and most often these foods are tampered with in some way. Gluten-related disorders are on the rise and increasing numbers of people are turning to a gluten-free diet to overcome a variety of signs and symptoms.

Beyond diagnosed coeliac disease and non-coeliac gluten sensitivity, there are three reasons I believe a gluten-free lifestyle is optimal:

1. Wheat is not what it used to be.
2. Gluten is indigestible.
3. Gluten is pro-inflammatory.

Diabetes and inflammatory digestive conditions continue to rise and increasing numbers of people want to eat for better health, more energy and improved mood.

Beyond diabetes and inflammatory digestive conditions, there are three reasons I would encourage you to follow a sugar free lifestyle:

1. Added sugar creates imbalance.
2. Fructose is addictive.
3. Reduced risk for inflammation.

Consumption of dairy products has also been linked to higher risk for cardiovascular disease, diabetes and various cancers, especially to cancers of the reproductive system.

You may need to consider a dairy free lifestyle, knowing

1. Milk naturally contains hormones and growth factors.
2. Non-organic milk contains contaminants.
3. To reduce mucous in the body and reduce inflammation, avoid dairy.

If you choose to explore these topics further, you can find out more in Nourish Well in *Section 9 - Your body - your vehicle for life* of the Resources chapter.

Move more

The health benefits of regular movement and physical activity are hard to ignore, particularly for the quality of your sleep and detoxification. Your immune system works in conjunction with your lymphatic system and the lymphatic system does not have a pump to move lymph through the body. For those of us dealing with chronic health challenges, it is critical to keep moving the lymph so that the toxins can be eliminated from the liver and kidneys.

Lauren Gelman wrote that movement is medicine for the mind and I agree. Physical activity makes your brain better by

1. boosting brain-building hormones like BDNF (Brain-derived neurotrophic factor) to 'fertilise the brain',
2. improving your brain's executive function, even with thirty minutes movement a day, in as little as four weeks,
3. stabilising your blood sugar after you eat, which protects you against insulin resistance and cognitive decline.

Focus on getting moving to release endorphins, which offset the stress hormones. This will reduce the effects of stress, anxiety and depression, in turn supporting you to have more restful sleep and improving your sense of well-being.

See everyday activities as a good opportunity to be active and increase the opportunity for social contact by doing physical activity with others.

Where to begin

If you are very ill, the best place to start is a graded exercise program. Your medical doctor can refer you to a physiotherapist or exercise physiologist to supervise you.

I researched graded exercise programs and recognised that for me personally, it was common sense:

1. Start small and where you are at right now.
2. Listen to your body and notice what feels right for you.
3. Move within your constraints yet slowly push the boundary.
4. As your stamina improves add a little more activity, but not so much that it will exacerbate your symptoms.

My starting point was dry brushing my skin before a bath or a few simple stretches to get my body moving and the muscles working. As I felt stronger I incorporated a walk on my driveway. My next step was to drive myself to the beach and park where I could walk to the nearby bench. Over time I made it down to the beach and began walking a short distance barefoot, knowing I had to get myself back to the car. As I felt ready I would increase the distance a little more.

Ready for your next step

As you build up your stamina I encourage you to also include incidental exercise into your day like

- dancing to music you love to add some fun,
- using the stairs and not the elevator,
- parking away from the entrance of the store, and

- if you are using public transport, get off a stop earlier and walk the rest of the way.

Any physical activity that uses breath work provides incredible benefits for your circulation, mood and overall well-being. The big plus is that it stimulates brain growth, even as we age. Also consider adding activities such as swimming (or even walking in the pool), restorative yoga, tai chi and qigong.

Remember to start slowly and pace yourself. I'd encourage you to research one of these practices on YouTube and follow a short session to see how you go. If you do decide to join a class, be sure to let the instructor know of your situation so they can tailor your routine.

Rest and recover

Sleep is the elixir of life and it is my belief that the quality of your sleep determines the quality of your life. Are you aware that sleep deprivation has the same impact as being drunk? Your decision-making is poorer, you are less productive and creative and to add more insult to injury, your waistline expands.

I researched everything I could about quality sleep and was amazed that putting in place simple rituals, such as a wind down to sleep, could have such a profound effect. The more consistent I was, the more my body's biology took over, and I began to be able to fall asleep easily, stay asleep all night, go back to sleep easily if woken and wake without an alarm.

The challenge when you are sleep-deprived is that you fall asleep from sheer exhaustion, but you don't sleep deeply or stay asleep. Before you know it, in the wee hours of the morning, your mind is racing around with 'to do's', 'what if's' and more.

Has sleep become a nasty playground?

The fears and worries we don't acknowledge in our waking life come out to play in the middle of the night. And it can be so nasty - worse than two kids having a spat in the playground.

Our mind gets stuck on auto-repeat and, like clockwork, it's two or three in the morning and we're wide awake, with the merry-go-round of thoughts swirling in our heads relentlessly.

We ruminate on things.

"If only I said…"
"How dare they…"
"I forgot to…"
"What if [fill in the blank] happens…"
"Will I make a fool of myself when …"

They could be conversations, events, plans and the like. Things that have happened, things that may or may not happen or things that are coming up are prime targets for repetition.

But what if there was another way? Imagine you could fall asleep and rest easily all through the night. How would that feel?

All your fears and worries need a space to surface, and so we need to give them their play time long before we head to bed.

It is completely possible to fall asleep and stay asleep when we understand that the mind makes a good slave but a poor master. If this sounds true for you, there is more on this in the next chapter *Your mind - a playground for thoughts.*

When you experience quality sleep, you are better equipped during the day to cope with life's stressors, and in turn this will support you to let go of ruminating at night.

I conducted a Sleep Quality Poll where thirty-seven percent of people said they still wake up tired even after a 'good' sleep. Can you imagine the impact of more than one third of people in your waking life being sleep deprived?

This was my story and I know that while sleep may not seem very sexy, you may not appreciate the tangible benefits of good sleep until you experience them.

How to get your Zzz's on in 8 key steps

1. Make sleep a priority in your life. It's about quality of sleep, not only quantity.
2. Disconnect from electronic devices at least one to two hours before going to bed. Ok you may have FOMO (Fear Of Missing Out) but give it a go.
3. Simulate dusk in your home. Use low wattage warm coloured light bulbs in lamps, not overhead lights.
4. Create a pre-sleep routine. A few personal rituals sending strong signals to the body that it's time for sleep, about thirty to sixty minutes before bed, is ideal.
5. Have a regular sleep-wake schedule. Your body is governed by a set of bio-rhythms, so work with them.
6. Create a sleep haven. A cool, darkened room, free of electronic devices and clutter.

7. Minimise likely disturbances to your sleep. Friendly chat to the neighbour about their dog or cat, maybe?
8. Keep a sleep diary. Get insights into any habits or patterns that impact your sleep and seek support for ongoing problems.

Power naps

People often ask me about napping during the day. When you're ill it is wise to let go of 'pushing through' and honour your body with a power nap (or two) instead. Aim for no more than thirty to forty-five minutes so you don't wake up in the middle of a sleep cycle and feel groggy. Be sure to take your power nap before 2pm during the day so it won't impact your night routine.

When I am doing work that requires new thinking, I still need to nap. It recharges my brain, allowing time for integration, and on waking I can continue with less taxing tasks.

If you need support with your sleep, head to *Rest and Recover* in *Section 9 - Your body - your vehicle for life* of the Resources chapter.

Take action

Pick one of these actions and focus on creating a new habit. When you feel you are on track then pick another action. This way you will avoid any overwhelm.

• Make a list of food-like substances you currently eat and what organic whole foods you will crowd these out with.

- Calculate how much pure water you will need to drink for well-being.
- Measure out your daily requirement of pure water and aim to drink most of it by midday.
- Review your eating protocol to determine whether removing inflammatory foods is optimal for you.
- Make a list of everyday and fun activities that are a good opportunity to be active within your constraints.
- Review the 8 key steps to quality sleep and decide what to implement going forward.

Your mind - a playground for thoughts

*Remembering that life is a journey allows us to lighten up on the
self-criticism and use our new perspective on previous experiences
as information to help us create a more loving,
accepting and brighter future*
Jarl Forsman and Steve Sekhon

Overview

I share this information with you so that you can create
sound mental health. We'll explore why the mind makes a
poor master and how to interrupt automatic ways of
thinking.

What you will find in this chapter are ideas for calming your
mind and creating alternative ways of being within yourself.

A calm mind influences the immune system positively,
whereas stress hormones have a negative impact that
compromise your body's ability to heal itself.

To get the most out of this chapter, once again I
recommend you be open to the possibilities of doing
different things AND doing things differently.

3 reasons why your mind makes a poor master

#1 Our mind has a role in keeping us safe

There is a part of the brain that is aimed at protecting us but
can be hypervigilant for the wrong reasons. While we may
be evolved in many ways, our brain can still have us locked
in fight, flight or freeze mode. When we are fearful, this part

of the brain is over-active and misinterprets signals from the environment, based on past experience or meanings we have previously attributed.

For example, you get an email that someone important to you or your business needs to talk to you urgently. What's your first reaction?

#2 Our perception of things is naturally blinkered

If there was an apple on the table and you viewed it from the front, it may look a certain way. Perhaps it was shiny with no blemishes. You may hold the perception that the apple was safe to eat as it is. However, if you viewed it from the back and saw a black spot, and on closer examination a worm was making its home there, you'd hold a different perception.

So it is with our perception of situations. We each have the capacity to take in information, but we do this in diverse ways because of the way we think.

The four thinking lenses we use on the same situation are

1. Logic,
2. Emotion,
3. Big-picture, and
4. Detailed.

And we generally prefer one or more to the others. This is how differences in perspectives of the same event arise.

Amplifying our perception of a situation is what can create unnecessary worry or fear, and yet it may be a blinkered version of the story.

#3 We label our emotions good or bad

You may have been conditioned from childhood that certain emotions were good or bad. A common one is that feeling angry is unacceptable, so instead of healthfully expressing ourselves, we internalise our feelings. This creates internal stress in the body and can manifest in physical and mental symptoms.

Finding a way to be ok with all emotions is possible and can be learned. As Petrea King, CEO of Quest for Life Foundation, says, "You are not your feelings, you have feelings".

Thoughts become us

Both Lao Tzu and Mahatma Ghandi are quoted on the connection between our thoughts, words, actions and habits. Given Lao Tzu was a Chinese philosopher in ancient times it may have been poetic licence by Mahatma Ghandi that he added beliefs becoming thoughts. Both concluded with habits becoming values or character, and therefore your destiny.

This is not a book on philosophy, however there is a strong link between your thoughts, words, actions and habits. There is a field of practice called Mind Body Medicine, which integrates the mind with the physical and energetic bodies for this very reason.

In the chapter *Explore the road to here*, I referenced two terms that I choose to use to create a distinction between unhelpful and helpful thoughts. They are 'stinky' thinking versus 'fragrant' thinking. Explore how heavy or light these juxtaposed thoughts make you feel.

To illustrate this, here are a few examples.

'Stinky' Thinking	'Fragrant' Thinking
The doctors say there is no cure, I won't get better	Today I will focus my energy on what I can do that is within my control
Nobody understands what it's like to be dealing with [fill in the blank]	Everyone has a story and I am rewriting mine one sentence at a time
I should / would / could have…	I'm grateful I'm learning as I go. I will find what works best for me
If only…	Today I choose to…

If you find yourself wading in 'stinky' thinking, be gentle with yourself. Capture your most common or recurring thoughts and rewrite them as 'fragrant' thoughts. Over time, as you put this into practice, you will transform automatic negative thoughts into more positive ones.

Reflect on where there is fear or anxiety and if required, go back to the exercises from the chapter *Explore the road to here* and redo these.

Frame of reference

Reframing an event as an impartial observer is another wonderful technique to use. When an event happens, we assign it meaning through our frame of reference, i.e. our thoughts, beliefs, values and patterns. With reframing, you can choose to change the way you look at something and consequently change how you experience it by finding a more constructive interpretation of what is happening to you.

This takes practise, patience and skill, so seek the support of a psychotherapist or psychologist if you find yourself unable to see other perspectives on your situation.

Mind your language

This is not about cussing or swearing, although that could be the truth of it too. Our mind doesn't discern between thoughts or the spoken word, so what we keep thinking or saying out loud, the brain takes literally. For example, if you are to constantly say, "I'm so stupid, anyone could do that", the mind reinforces the words you're saying as a form of negative conditioning that can lead to a downward spiral.

Negative self-talk is a barrier to good mental health, so we need to be willing to bring to the surface, explore and create a positive space in our language as a part of our well-being journey.

A different example you may have experienced is when your brain skips over a word in a sentence that begins with a double negative. For example, "Don't forget to take your tablets". The brain interprets this as, "Forget to take your tablets". So, what's the action you need to take? Substituting the above for the positive statement, "Remember to take your tablets" is an easy fix.

Focus on building awareness of how you use language and work on switching out the automatic negative responses with more loving, kind responses and put your inner mean girl or boy back in their box.

Herding cats

Our stray thoughts are really like many cats wandering around, scattering what precious focus you have. But there are several ways that can be helpful to calm your mind and body:

1. Breath work.
2. Full body relaxation.
3. Guided or Self-led Meditation.

If you have a crazy busy mind like me, you may wonder how you can possibly do any of these? My suggestion is to begin with the breath because it's portable, accessible and it truly works.

Breath work

Your breath is a tool that you have in every moment and in every situation. Your breath can calm the sympathetic nervous system and take you out of fight, flight or freeze mode. By using your breath consciously and mindfully, you can shift into a calm state quickly.

One technique I teach my clients is Dr Andrew Weil's 4-7-8 breath. It's simple:

1. Place the tip of the tongue on the roof of your mouth and keep it there.
2. Exhale with a whooshing sound through your mouth.
3. Breathe in through your nostrils for four counts.

4. Hold your breath for seven counts.
5. Release the breath with a whooshing sound through your mouth for eight counts.
6. Repeat steps 3 - 5 four times once a day to begin with, and then use twice a day for maintenance or when required.

I incorporate this type of breath work when I go for a walk in nature, this ensures I am beginning my walk by relieving my body of any pent-up anxiety or stress.

Another technique I find useful is alternate nostril breathing, a Yogic practice. It balances the hemispheres of the brain and supports the connection of mind and body. It takes practise to do this effortlessly however the mind is occupied with what to do not your stress, and the benefits are immense.

If your right hand is dominant

1. Begin by using the thumb of your right hand to close your right nostril.
2. Breathe in gently through your left nostril.
3. Place your middle finger on your left nostril and, releasing your thumb, exhale gently through your right nostril.
4. Breathe in gently through your right nostril.
5. Place your thumb on your right nostril and, releasing your middle finger, exhale gently through your left nostril.
6. Repeat for a few rounds.

If your left hand is dominant, simply switch hands and reverse the process.

You will find more information and links to videos on these practices in *Section 10 - Your mind - a playground for thoughts* of the Resources chapter.

Full body relaxation

I first learned the power of full body relaxation when I did a Mindfulness Based Stress Reduction (MBSR) course, founded by Dr Jon Kabat-Zinn at University of Massachusetts Medical School. In the eight-week course, we did what they refer to as a body scan. In my layman's terms, this involves bringing attention to each part of the body, as you would do in the practice of Yoga Nidra. What was so helpful was that in the process of being guided to focus on a body part, being curious and exploring what's going on and breathing into it, my mind chatter was turned off.

When I incorporated this into my bedtime wind down routine, I noticed that sleeping peacefully at night was a given. However, the point of the body scan is not to fall asleep. Yet I found as I gave myself permission to do what my body needed most at the time, it worked much better for me.

No angst. No stress. Pure bliss.

The *Calm and Collected* audio from my website can be downloaded and saved on your smartphone so you can do this practice as the need arises. You can find this and a link to a free online MBSR course in *Section 10 - Your mind - a playground for thoughts* of the Resources chapter.

Self-led or guided meditation

Are you still not convinced that meditation is for you, even despite all the media attention on the benefits? That's ok, I understand, because I was where you are now.

My podcast guest, Dr Kathy Gruver had a great technique she shared with listeners who felt they couldn't meditate. It involved these six simple steps:

1. Choose a state you'd like to feel, e.g. calm and peaceful.
2. Find a quiet space where you won't be interrupted.
3. Close your eyes gently.
4. On your in breath, mentally say the words, "I am".
5. On your out breath, mentally say the words, "calm and peaceful".
6. Keep doing this until you're ready to open your eyes.

How easy is that? You can do this anytime you need to, for however long you choose.

My positive experience with meditation happened when I attended one of *Quest for Life Foundation*'s residential programs. Several times across the day we would get ourselves comfortable on the floor or in a chair and would be led in a guided meditation with voice and music. I experienced an inordinate amount of calm, peace and clarity that I hadn't before. I had believed that my mind was too busy to meditate. But I found that the more I let go of the notion of 'perfecting' meditation, the easier it became to be still with my thoughts, with curiosity not judgement.

Given this positive experience, I purchased Petrea King's meditation CDs. My favourites to this day are Rainbows to Heal meditations. One is for self-healing and another for extending healing to others. Petrea King shaped my healing journey in a very practical, lasting way and I'm so grateful to her and the *Quest for Life Foundation.*

Sometimes, finding someone whose voice or approach you connect with can be a challenge. You want to be feeling calm instead of irritated. If you feel the need for guided meditation, my recommendation is to use the *Insight Timer* app for smartphones. There are several meditation teachers who have free meditations. My favourites are those by Tom Evans, also my podcast guest. His voice is so calming, and his humour makes for a fabulous experience. Find more information in *Section 10 - Your mind - a playground for thoughts* of the Resources chapter.

Take action

- Capture your most common or recurring thoughts and rewrite them as 'fragrant' thoughts.
- Reflect on where there is fear or anxiety and if required, go back to the exercises from the chapter *Explore the road to here* and redo these.
- Focus on building awareness of how you use language and work on switching out the automatic negative responses.
- Select a breath practice and make this part of your daily routine:
  o Practice Dr Andrew Weil's 4-7-8 breath twice a day.
  o Use alternative nostril breathing to support the connections of mind and body.
- Select a restorative practice and make this part of your daily routine

Your soul - the essence guiding you

*You were put on this earth to achieve your greatest self,
to live out your purpose, and to do it courageously.*
Steve Maraboli

Overview

I share this information with you so that you will seize the opportunity to create holistic health and well-being by integrating body, mind and soul.

What you will find in this chapter are ideas for creating meaning in your life and finding pleasure that nurtures and feeds your soul. For me the soul is the essence and spirit of me that will journey on after my physical body leaves this world.

So, I experience soulfulness as the purpose and meaning for my life and as true connection with others. There's no doubt for me that there is something greater than myself at work. This belief builds hope and resilience, as I don't believe anyone would choose to be chronically ill.

I believe that when you uncover what your purpose is, and you create meaning for your life, it helps you to cope with the physical experience of your health challenges.

To get the most out of this chapter, be open to the possibility that this is your time to be who you truly are and to find your true north.

Shining your light on purpose

Even though you're feeling ill, you need a daily purpose to create meaning in your life. Even if you feel you have lost sight of the possibilities for your future on the all-consuming journey back to well-being and that your body has let you down, I believe your soul purpose awaits.

You can focus on what your purpose is for this time, even if you can't see clearly to the end of your days. At this time, your purpose doesn't need to be grand like Oprah Winfrey's.

For me, writing this book has been one of the most enriching and cathartic experiences of my well-being journey. It's made meaning out of this roller coaster ride of being ill for so long. In the process I have recognised that my purpose is to enable others to see the possibilities for their life and make a difference by speaking out and being an advocate for those with an invisible chronic illness.

I've been an educator for much of my life, so this book is the beginning of me fulfilling this purpose. However, if you had asked me four years ago, I would not have even conceived of writing a self-help book for people who, like me, are dealing with chronic health challenges.

Uncovering your purpose is not about waiting for perfect phrasing, perfect timing or perfect health and well-being. It is the ability to create meaning in your life where you're at right now, by being connected with others and of service in some way every day.

When you know what your purpose is, you can wake up each day and live it, so we're going to shine a light on what your purpose is, where you are at right now.

My friend and colleague, Tracy Otsuka believes that we come into this world with an internal GPS that is perfectly capable of guiding us to make great major life decisions. So, I enlisted her to share her process for living your purpose.

Here are the steps Tracy teaches when uncovering your purpose.

You don't find your purpose, you step into it

You often hear people talking about finding their purpose and this is where we get it wrong. Finding your purpose typically sends you outside yourself for the answers.

It makes everyone else the expert on your life, which pretty much guarantees that you'll be living their purpose instead of yours. Rather, go within yourself. The seeds of your purpose have been there since birth. Only you are capable of stepping into it. So how do you do that?

Find the feeling

Start with your childhood. When is the first time that you remember doing something or being somewhere where you knew you were in your zone of genius, doing exactly what you needed to be doing in that moment. You were lit up but calm, peaceful, and happy. How did this feel in your body? That is the feeling that being in the neighbourhood of your purpose elicits.

Now, think of a time when you just knew everything was wrong and you're certain that you weren't living your purpose. How did you feel this in your body? Were you anxious, overwhelmed? Did you feel heavy in your body?

Maybe that's exactly how you feel now. For reference, that is exactly how you do not want to feel.

For some of you, this exercise may be difficult. You may remember very little about your childhood. Instead, ask yourself if there's something that happened in your childhood that provides the meaning today. It could be one kind person who took an interest in you, who recognised something special in you, who showed you who you could be.

If you can't come up with anything positive from your childhood, move on to other times in your life, starting with college or university, in your career, in relationships, working on a hobby, volunteering.

When did you first feel that 'lit-up from inside' feeling, that you were exactly where you should be in that moment? Once you can identify one of those feelings, then you can scan your life for other times that you felt that same feeling.

Get out your journal or grab a pen and paper and go through your life, starting from your childhood, and write down every 'lit up, I'm in my zone of genius, doing exactly what I should be doing' feeling that you can remember. Then highlight any themes that you might see. What do they have in common?

Do you see an overall pattern or a theme of nature, animals, people, movement, family? Purpose, after all, is just one of your passions that you've attached a side of service to. It's your unique way of helping people or contributing to a cause that's important to you and adding value. It's that simple.

Look for opportunities that really light you up and intersect with your passions but that are also in alignment with your values. That's the sweet spot, the neighbourhood where your purpose lives.

Giving meaning to your past

The best purposes are those that give meaning to your past. They explain why you had to go through what you went through. You're also now in a position, because of your past, where you're helping someone else not go through what you went through. It explains why you're here on this planet and puts your life in context.

It may also feel like something that was 'meant to happen', and you know this instinctively or intuitively. It takes you out of victim mode and gives you back your power; because suddenly you understand the reason why it was so important that this happened to you.

You can find out more about Tracy Otsuka and her work in *Section 11 - Your soul - the essence guiding you* of the Resources chapter.

A guiding framework

Our values create our own inner compass and now more than ever, when we live aligned with our values, we will feel integrated and whole. The English Oxford living dictionary defines values as "principles or standards of behaviour; one's judgement of what is important in life".

Values are what inform thoughts, words and action, and so guide our decisions and the resulting behaviour.

Two perspectives on our values

Individual values may include things such as fun, creativity, humility, honesty and health. When we live congruently with our individual values, it reflects with clarity what we prioritise in our decisions and the choices we make which ultimately create the future we need.

Relationship values may include things such as openness, trust, generosity, commitment, appreciation and kindness. These values inform our desire for connection with others, whether they are life partners, family, friends or work colleagues. Think of a time when you were your happiest or most satisfied in your work. There is a strong likelihood that your individual and relationship values were being met and they aligned with the associated organisation's values and norms.

For example, if honesty were an individual value for you, you would not be willing to work with an organisation that conducts business in an unethical way. Or, if you can recall a time when you were in some level of conflict with a friend or family member, it is highly likely that some of your personal and / or relationship values were not being met.

If punctuality is an individual value and your friend is repeatedly late, it will create friction unless you talk about it and find some middle ground.

Communicating your values is key to positive relationships with others, as we all have different values.

Values refresher

You may have had values that evolved based on your personal growth, so take time to reflect on your values at this life stage. If you are stuck for ideas on what your individual and relationship values are, you will find lists of words by searching for these terms online.

Here's a quick way to refresh your values:

- Aim to list about ten top individual and relationship values.
- Prioritise your top ten until you have no more than five values.
- List one main core value plus your other top four values.
- Test if these values are a good fit with your Intention.
- Next, ask yourself if you would be willing to uphold these even if you were different?

For example, if your main core value is honesty, you likely believe that the truth and doing the right thing matters greatly. When someone fabricates a story or attempts to deceive you, what will you do? Will you call them on their behaviour in a loving way, even if it means they may react badly? Will you share your opinion even if it differs from other viewpoints?

You may take another action to remain aligned to your values, however, for your top five values it is important that you would be willing to take a stand.

Use your five values to guide you and make the best choices for yourself, creating happiness and contentment in the process.

Soul pleasures

Have you ever stopped to think about what really lights you up? What gives you pleasure and a deep sense of joy? When

I was training as an integrative holistic well-being coach, we talked about secondary food (or the other aspects of our lives, beyond basic human needs, that we need to feel truly alive).

This is your relationship to self and others, your work, your contribution to a cause and your connection to a community, all of which make you feel enriched. I've already shared the need to surround yourself with positive people, enjoy positive relationships through upholding your values and boundaries, so those are a given.

We weren't designed to live in isolation, and nor are we designed to be without pleasure. While you've been dealing with your chronic health challenges you may have needed to let go of some of the things that made you feel joyful and warmed your soul. But it's now time to find out how you can participate within your constraints. Is there something you are willing to do on your own? Perhaps you feel the need to be in the company of others?

Make a list of attainable activities to bring more joy into your life, that you either do solo or can bring into a relationship or connection or contribution with others.

Here's a starter list for you:

- Smile at everyone you meet.
- Create a playlist of your favourite uplifting music.
- Dance as if nobody's watching.
- Sit outdoors and listen to the sounds of nature.
- Walk along the beach barefoot.
- Watch a sunrise or sunset.
- Enjoy mindful colouring in or a paint by number picture.

- Lose yourself in a delightful book, paper based or audio.
- Learn a new craft or hobby.
- Learn how to cook a new dish.
- Offer to teach someone a skill that's second nature to you.
- Take a class in something that interests you.
- Join the local library and participate in some free events.
- Find a local community project where you can volunteer your time.
- Find a cause that you believe in and see what support you can offer.
- Watch a feel-good movie or your favourite movie again.
- Call a friend and commit to talking about anything but your health.
- Arrange a catch-up with a friend.
- Play with or be around young children for a fun injection.
- Take a photo of everything beautiful you see and share them with others.

Use your attainable activities list as a prompt each day so that you are acting on and building up your soul pleasures.

Take action

- Complete the activity to uncover your purpose.
- Complete the values refresher and communicate these to people who matter to you.
- Make a list of attainable activities to bring more joy into your life, that you either do solo or can bring into a relationship or connection or contribution with others.

Taking back your personal power

If you're interested you'll do what's convenient; if you're committed you'll do whatever it takes.
John Assaraf

Overview

I share this information with you because you do have the freedom to choose. In every moment of every day, choice is yours.

You need something different for your life. You are making the choice that life doesn't need to be lived defined by a chronic illness or dis-ease. You are far more resilient than you know.

It's the everyday steps that you take that will bring about profound change in your health and well-being. It's not the big silver bullet that people are often waiting for. Every choice you make towards your Intention is what's going to get you there.

What you will find in this chapter are ideas for you to get clear on how to move forward, with this new understanding of yourself, and with your desire for well-being. You will have clarity on the opportunities for your well-being despite the diagnosis you have.

We will explore how to build new habits, taking small consistent steps towards what we need, rather than what we don't want.

To get the most out of this chapter, remind yourself that there is always possibility. The possibility of what your well-being journey may look like, going forward from today. As well as the possibility that things will be different, and you have the opportunity to enjoy your evolution on the way.

Decide what you're committed to and make this your priority. I believe when you make a commitment and put your energy and focus on this, it is both possible and achievable. The universe will conspire with you to make that happen.

Our focus is shifting from 'knowing' to 'being and embodying'. Knowing what to do, or simply having knowledge, is useless on its own. We need to move that knowing forward into being. Become a human being instead of a human doing. More being, less doing.

The past doesn't define you or your future. As I have noted before, you have arrived at this place of ill-health and you are on a journey. Taking back your personal power is within your control. You can make the choices, take small and consistent steps, and use these to move your well-being forward each day.

Exercising your choice

For the next set of activities, you will need four blank pieces of A4 or Letter size paper. These could be in an exercise book or loose pages.

Review what you wrote as your Intention from the chapter *Begin with the end in mind*. Explore that against your Stocktake from the chapter *Explore the road to here* as well as where you are now with your well-being.

Look at this from two aspects.

1. Why do you need to move forward to your desired Intention?
2. What is it that you need for your well-being?

Within you, you have an awareness between the current and future state for your well-being. You have ideas from working through this book. You have an inner knowing of what you need. You may have even tried something before, but were inconsistent, so did not realise results.

Now is a good time to refresh your understanding of the I.AM model from the chapter *Explore the road to here*.

On your first piece of paper, create three columns. In column one, write a list of all the things you need to action to close the gap between where you are now and where you need to be with your well-being.

At this time, you are brainstorming. Write down every possible action or step you could take, without passing judgement on whether it's feasible or achievable at this time.

Keep writing, and when you feel you can't write anymore, take a break and then come back to it and write some more.

Now, in the second column, add which of the four aspects; mental, physical, emotional and soulful, each step or action supports. Some may straddle more than one of these aspects and that is good news.

Observe the proportion of the four aspects. Is this balanced between the four aspects? If not, top up the aspects that are low.

The next step is to ask yourself this question, "What am I ready, willing and able to do?"

- Within the next twenty-four hours.
- Within the next week.
- Within four weeks.
- Within eight weeks.
- Within twelve weeks.

Write your responses in column three. This is the basis of your Commitment Plan at a high level. The aim is to work in twelve-week blocks, so you can test, review and pivot your choices as necessary.

Making a commitment

The next step is making a commitment that is realistic, motivating and supports you. What obstacles do you see that would stop you from exercising your choice?

On a second piece of paper create two columns. Get clarity by writing down in column one, all the obstacles and objections that come up. In column two, write down all the counter arguments to each obstacle and objection.

If you can't overcome an obstacle, can you set that choice aside for now?

Are you somebody who over commits and then feels overwhelmed? If so, what choice(s) can you set aside for the following 12-week block? What are your concerns with putting these choices into action?

On the third piece of paper make three columns. In the first column, write down all your concerns and fears. Explore whether these are arising because you are taking yourself out of your comfort zone. What evidence is there that this concern is real at this time? What fears may be realised as you exercise your choice?

In the second column, write down what the likelihood is of them happening – extreme, medium, high, low. In the third column, write down what the potential negative impact on your well-being would be – extreme, medium, high, low.

This will highlight that even though something is extremely likely to happen, its impact may be low. The inverse is also feasible, where the negative impact is extremely high and yet the likelihood is low.

Your appetite for taking calculated risks will help you recognise how far you are willing to push outside of your comfort zone. Sit with this in contemplation and, if necessary, journal your thoughts to release any fears.

What is within your control and what is not? Your Commitment Plan needs to contain choices that are within your control. The graded exercise program that was discussed earlier is a good example. If you made a choice to be walking 10,000 steps a day in twelve weeks, when you can barely walk to the end of the driveway, that wouldn't be realistic. The impact on your well-being may be high or extreme. However, walking 1,000 steps a day, consistently by four weeks, may be achievable.

Because of these reflections, do you need to re-calibrate your first 12-week Commitment Plan?

Your Commitment Plan

At this point, you are now ready to write your Commitment Plan. On a fourth piece of paper make three columns. In the first column, write down the choices that you will exercise in the timeframe you opted for. To shift your Commitment

Plan into being, have clarity on how the changes you are proposing to make will lead to your Intention.

In the second column of your Commitment Plan, make a note of how each change you need to make supports your Intention. This will reinforce your commitment and keep you on the path to your Intention.

In the third column of your Commitment Plan, write a completion date for the choice you are exercising.

You now have a very tangible way of making the changes you need for your well-being. Every three months, come back to this process so you can check off your progress on your original list of ideas and potentially add new ones. Continuing like this in 12-week blocks will build the momentum that you need to exercise all your choices for your well-being.

For help with this activity head to www.hopeinadarktunnel.com to download your free guidebook.

Consistent action over perfection

When creating new habits, aim for consistency not perfection. We are human and fallible, so give yourself grace that even the best laid plans may not experience one hundred percent success. However, executing your Commitment Plan to eighty percent each day would have you achieve far more than if you had never started.

Rewiring for healthy habits requires simple, repeatable, achievable steps done with consistency. You need to be organised and prepared to be sure you will realise your Commitment Plan.

On a Sunday, take time to review what you have committed to for the week. Put the actions in your diary or planner and place it somewhere visible.

I think the refrigerator is a fabulous place for your weekly commitment because every time you go there you remind your brain what you're doing, and that helps you stay on track.

To build accountability, share your weekly commitment with someone who cares for you and is willing to check in with how you went. Find someone who celebrates your wins, doesn't judge and asks questions about what obstacles stopped you from doing what you needed to.

By being organised and taking steps each week, these new habits will create neural pathways in the brain, which will make them automatic over time.

Give yourself some grace, remembering that new habits take time to build. There's a school of thought that it takes 28 days to form a new habit. However, that could be limiting if it's something that's really a big stretch for you.

When it comes to your physical health, you need to plan your meals ahead, then shop and prepare for the week so that you've got everything you need in the refrigerator. No room for excuses, only possibilities.

For your graded exercise program, you may choose to enlist a friend. By doing physical movement with someone you have the social aspect added to it, plus accountability.

Another way to feel prepared for our mental and emotional health activities is to allocate them a time in the day when you'll do them. Don't leave it up to chance. Ensure that it's in your diary or your planner, whatever you choose to use, just make sure to set aside the time.

With my meditation or full body relaxation, the easiest way for me to make sure I did them was to associate them with waking and before I go to bed. That's quite specific and it means that I now do it. It's not a question of if I've got time; it's simply part of my daily routine.

The other key to consistency is to aim for fun and pleasure. When we add novelty, our brain absolutely loves it, so it supports us right back. We are looking for ways to feed our soul, and so making things fun and pleasurable lifts our joy and our feel-good factor.

What are the ways that you can think of to make any of your choices more fun? Is it that you add something (like music) to things that you don't normally enjoy? For example, perhaps you're not a Cordon Bleu chef, so putting on your music playlist while you cook will give you the opportunity to feel positive and high vibe. In the process, you may learn to love cooking.

You can take back your personal power and reclaim well-being one step at a time. I believe in you and your infinite possibility. You can do this!

Take action

- Review your Intention (future state) and your Stocktake (current state).
- Write a list of all the things you need to action to close the gap between where you are now and where you need to be with your well-being.

- Add which of the four aspects; mental, physical, emotional and soulful, each step or action supports.
- Observe the proportion of the four aspects and top up aspects that are low.
- Allocate a timeframe to each step or action.
- Write down all the obstacles and objections that come up.
- Write down all the counter arguments to each obstacle and objection.
- Write down all your concerns and fears.
- Write down what the likelihood is of them happening – extreme, medium, high, low.
- Write down what the potential negative impact on your well-being would be – extreme, medium, high, low.
- Reflect on all these activities and re-calibrate as appropriate.
- Create your 12-week Commitment Plan focusing on the choices that you will exercise in the timeframe you opted for, how each change supports your Intention and a completion date.
- On a Sunday, take time to review what you have committed to for the week.
- Put the actions in your diary or planner and place it somewhere visible.
- Every three months, come back to this process so you can check off your progress on your original list of ideas and potentially add new ones.

Coming back to you

To be beautiful means to be yourself. You don't need to be
accepted by others. You need to accept yourself.
Thich Nhat Hanh

Overview

I share this information with you because your choices
create your future. You are amazing and unique the way you
are right now and your body, mind and soul desire
something more for you than chronic health challenges.

Lifelong learning is the key to your ongoing well-being. We
need to be creating the space for ourselves where learning
and growing is part of our everyday being.

What you'll find in this chapter are ideas for you to explore
so that you can show up as your vibrant, beautiful self,
harness each and every opportunity, and prioritise lifelong
learning.

To get the most out of this chapter you need to believe that
life isn't perfect, and nor are we. We previously explored
how taking imperfect and consistent action is far more
beneficial for you than staying stuck where you are.

To keep evolving on your journey, get clear on your
priorities for your life and for your well-being. We are not
arriving at a destination and unpacking, we are on a journey.

Are you going to do different things AND do things
differently?

How do you want to show up?

Do you love all of yourself? Have you reached the point of self-acceptance that encompasses everything about yourself? Perhaps you don't love a physical attribute. Do you think your derrière is too large, your nose too prominent or perhaps you think your hair is not thick enough? Loving all of yourself requires self-love, self-validation and self-compassion.

Self-love

Self-love is reaching the point where you recognise that this is the body you were given. It's perfectly imperfect. There is more to life than spending time concerning yourself with physical attributes that you can do nothing about.

I'm not judging you if you decided to have cosmetic surgery, it may have been in your highest and best good. However, women, and nowadays more men, feel external pressure to look a certain way.

Ask what is it that you don't love about yourself? How can you bring conscious awareness to it? Contemplate what would help you to move forward from those thoughts.

Act as if you love yourself. Only you can make a choice to move forward and love yourself unconditionally. Over time, you will recognise that all parts of you are designed to be uniquely you. They are all parts of you that are totally acceptable as they are.

With social media, I observe that people are judging their contribution or worth by how many likes or comments that they get on their Facebook business page or their personal pages. What if you just showed up as yourself every day and shared your wisdom from a place of self-love and self-acceptance?

Self-validation

We often look to others to validate that we are enough and that we are acceptable as we are. We constantly ask other's opinions, not making a decision of our own accord.

Self-validation involves accepting your own inner observation, your thoughts and your feelings. Use mindfulness to explore what you are experiencing and be curious about thoughts and feelings.

So, how can we validate ourselves? One way is to catch yourself doing fabulous things and reward yourself for doing them. Positive reinforcement grows confidence. Another way is to gather the facts, reflect on them and decide. Trust your inner wisdom and embodied knowledge. If the outcome isn't what you want, review what is required and pivot.

Remember, we are perfectly imperfect, and learning from our mistakes leads to personal growth and resilience.

Self-compassion

The compassion that you show for others needs to be shown to yourself too. When we make mistakes, it serves to remind us of how human we are. Self-compassion is when something has not gone to plan, but you have understanding and empathy for yourself in that moment. Be kinder to yourself so that self-compassion becomes a natural way of being.

Loving yourself takes ongoing practise. It's a way of being. It's something that you nurture every day. On days when you feel self-critical, accept that it's only for now and have self-compassion.

Your authentic self

Showing up as your authentic self every day ensures that you are living in alignment with who you truly are. There is congruence to your thoughts, your feelings, your words and your actions. It means showing up authentically whether you are behind closed doors, with friends, with family or with colleagues. You are creating your legacy.

I love Maya Angelou's quote: "At the end of the day people won't remember what you said or did, they will remember how you made them feel."

What do you want to be known for?

Shape your future

Where are you in your priority queue? Do you consistently put your needs to the back of the queue? This was me, and even now, sometimes it can start to slip. When I catch myself and focus on my Intention to be well, that is what brings me back to giving priority to what I want most.

Stephen R. Covey, author of *The 7 Habits of Highly Effective People*, talked about time management as a way of honouring your most important priorities. His example was filling a beaker with different materials that you'd find on a beach. He equated big rocks to the most important things in your life, i.e. the highest priorities. Your health and well-being, your family time, physical movement, social needs and aspects of your personal development could all potentially fit here.

Covey also had small pebbles, which were important life aspects, but not the highest in priority. And then he had sand. Sand represented the things we are called upon to do as part of our daily life, our obligations.

When he filled the beaker with sand and tried to fit in the pebbles and big rocks, it didn't work. He could not fit each of those three elements in. However, when he placed the big rocks in the beaker first, followed by some pebbles and then filled the beaker with the sand, all three elements fitted in with ease. He demonstrated that if we ignore our priorities and act on whatever seems urgent and not important, we won't have time for our big rocks.

What change would you make when planning, to set your highest priorities first?

Focusing on your highest priorities

The simplest way is to take your diary or your electronic calendar and set repeating appointments for things that matter most and are your highest priority. Block them out at a time of day that suits the activity or the intention. Your big rocks need to be non-negotiable.

As I've mentioned before, a big rock for me is starting and ending my day with contemplation and meditation. It has enabled me to sleep better, to show up more focused each day and to manage my stress despite any chronic health challenges.

Another big rock for me is to nourish my body deeply. One practical way I do this is going to the Sunday farmers markets. I buy fresh organic whole foods and have no excuse during the week not to complete my Commitment Plan and realise the Intention for my well-being.

What about time for socialising? Is it a big rock or a pebble? We know that social interaction is vital for our well-being, so plan something that's within your constraints. It could be as simple as keeping an hour or two free once or twice a week and deciding what to do on the day.

You may choose to connect and interact with someone in person or via phone. When you're creating an opportunity to connect with that person, hear what they have to share and, equally importantly, share what's going on for you. When you're in a place of being ill it can be easy to focus on what's not working in your life. My guidance is to start your conversation with, "What's new and good in your world?" This gives you both the opportunity to share things you are grateful for and sets the tone for the conversation.

We've explored how your thoughts influence your behaviour, the choices you make, as well as the decisions, and therefore the actions, you take. So, moment by moment you are creating and shaping your future. Choose wisely.

You have everything you need within yourself to move forward and experience well-being. Now, notice I'm not talking about being in a one hundred percent dis-ease free state.

When we place priority and focus on our Intention for our health and well-being, in each moment we can make a choice for our highest and best good. I believe, in time and with the right conditions, the body has the resources to heal itself.

Keep growing

Our whole being revolves around evolution and personal growth. When you set a priority to learn new things, you will be developing your brain and adding to your social well-being all in one go. Have you ever taken a dance lesson? Perhaps you feel self-conscious? But why let that stop you from giving your brain and body a good workout, from having fun and from meeting new people. What about learning a hobby or craft, e.g. painting, sewing, baking? The list is endless.

One of my favourite activities is sculpting with clay. You get in the flow, with your hands covered in 'mud', and focus the mind on the here and now.

Our brain thrives when we include novelty and fun. Creating novelty gives the brain the opportunity to create new neural pathways. Instead of corrosion setting in, over time, those highways of information will be reinforced or have a new side street built.

Having fun and being playful is part of building up your joy bank. Anytime when you are feeling low in resilience, you can remind yourself how you feel when you take part in something that is fun. Laughter is one of the most amazing ways to lift your feel-good hormone, serotonin. Watching funny movies and having a good belly laugh is good for the soul and so is sharing those moments with friends.

To keep growing, be sure to continue adding ideas to your Commitment Plan. Test new things to see what works for you. Reframe what's not working and explore whether it's because you're out of your comfort zone or because something needs to pivot.

Take time to celebrate how far you've come. Remember your realistic measure of how much progress you've made and take time to acknowledge this. Keep challenging yourself to move out of your comfort zones.

My wish for you is that you will be living well and living fabulously every day. You are on the road to well-being, one consistent yet imperfect step at a time.

Take action

- Bring conscious awareness of what you don't love about yourself. Contemplate what would help you to move forward from those thoughts.
- Act as if you love yourself. Only you can make a choice to move forward and love yourself unconditionally.
- Catch yourself doing fabulous things and reward yourself for doing them.
- Gather the facts, reflect on them and decide. Trust your inner wisdom and embodied knowledge. If the outcome isn't what you want, review what is required and pivot.
- Be kinder to yourself so that self-compassion becomes a natural way of being.
- What change would you make when planning, to set your highest priorities first? Block them out at a time of day that suits the activity or the intention.
- What new hobby or craft could you learn?
- What fun and playful activities can you include that build up your joy bank?

Acknowledgements

There are so many people who provided encouragement and support along my journey and I am deeply grateful to each one of you.

Kandé and Timothy you have helped me weather the storm with your endless support and love. Thank you for all you do for me without exception and for giving me the grace to be imperfect and fallible.

Alexis and Evelyn, you are the light of Gogo's life and bring me so much joy. You have taught me the simplicity of heart-based soulful living through your innocence, curiosity and playfulness.

Denise, Noel and Sharon, you took me in and gave me shelter. Your act of kindness was beyond measure and I am deeply indebted to you.

Margaret, Roberta and Soness, you were my advocates when I could not speak up for myself. Your ongoing support and friendship is deeply appreciated.

Allison, Anne and Helen thank you for always believing in me and my mission. Your sound counsel, wisdom and friendship are invaluable.

Catherine and Leigh, I marvel at how your calls were so well timed and made me laugh at the world and myself when you called BS on things.

Jane, Karen and Kathy, you shaped my thinking and helped me take imperfect action to bring my book to life. Much gratitude to you.

Ilana I'm truly grateful for the many hours you spent reviewing my first manuscript. I treasure your ongoing support and friendship.

Assisi and Gary, your guidance in editorial have made me feel so proud of this book. Thank you for ensuring my message is clear.

To you the readers of this book I send this *Ancient Tibetan Buddhist Blessing*
May you all be filled with loving kindness
May you all be well
May you all be peaceful and at ease
May you all be happy

About the Author

Bev Roberts works with business women to transform their well-being by 'rewiring' to create healthy habits and lasting change. She is a certified well-being transformation specialist and holds a Master's Degree in Behavioural Change and Strategy.

Though chronic illness robbed Bev of a successful career as an award-winning board-certified executive and accredited master change leadership consultant, she reinvented herself and retrained her brain through her love of learning. Her approach to health and change draws on neuroplasticity and holistically integrates four facets of well-being - physical, mental, emotional and soulful.

Bev is an advocate for those with invisible chronic illnesses, a voice and champion for those needing the critical knowledge and language to change their circumstances despite their current condition. Courageous and vulnerable, Bev insightfully articulates her open-hearted, pragmatic message to empower all who need it.

Bev enjoys a quiet beachside lifestyle and is a Glam-ma to two beautiful granddaughters' who help her to stay curious, playful and joyful.

Connect with Bev online and find out more about her free resources and online services.

f	Livingfabulouslywithbev	🌐	livingfabulously.com
in	bevroberts	🐦	C_Change

References

Angelou, M., n.d. *Good Reads.* [Online]
Available at:
https://www.goodreads.com/author/show/3503.Maya_An
gelou
[Accessed April 2018].

Assaraf, J., 2014. *AZ Quotes.* [Online]
Available at: http://www.azquotes.com/author/63396-
John_Assaraf
[Accessed April 2018].

Covey, S. R., 2013. *The 7 Habits of Highly Effective People.*
London: Simon & Schuster Ltd.

Dictionary, E. O. L., n.d. *English Oxford Living Dictionary.*
[Online]
Available at:
https://en.oxforddictionaries.com/definition/value
[Accessed April 2018].

Forsman, J. & Sekhon, S., 2005 - 2018. *Gratitude 24 x 7,* s.l.:
s.n.

Gelman, L., n.d. *Readers Digest.* [Online]
Available at: https://www.rd.com/health/fitness/6-ways-
exercise-makes-your-brain-better/
[Accessed April 2018].

Gruver, D. K., 2018. *Living Fabulously.* [Online]
Available at: https://www.livingfabulously.com/podcast-
archives/2018/1/8/061-are-you-doing-your-being-dr-kathy-
gruver
[Accessed April 2018].

Hanh, T. N., n.d. *Good Reads.* [Online]
Available at:
https://www.goodreads.com/work/quotes/959684-the-art-of-power
[Accessed April 2018].

Hyman, M., 2014. *Huff Post The Blog.* [Online]
Available at: https://www.huffingtonpost.com/dr-mark-hyman/chronic-disease_b_4221141.html
[Accessed April 2018].

Hyman, M., 2014. *Huff Post The Blog.* [Online]
Available at: https://www.huffingtonpost.com/dr-mark-hyman/diet-exercise_b_5482608.html
[Accessed April 2018].

Hyman, M., n.d. *AZ Quotes.* [Online]
Available at: http://www.azquotes.com/author/36883-Mark_Hyman_M_D
[Accessed April 2018].

King, P., n.d. *Wendy Mak.* [Online]
Available at: https://wendymak.com/top-ten-tips-avoid-anxiety-guest-blogger-petrea-king/
[Accessed April 2018].

Lipman, F., 2009. *Dr Frank Lipman's Daily Dose Blog.* [Online]
Available at: https://www.bewell.com/blog/why-we-need-to-change-the-health-care-system/
[Accessed April 2018].

Maraboli, S., n.d. *Good Reads.* [Online]
Available at:
https://www.goodreads.com/work/quotes/14708444-life-the-truth-and-being-free
[Accessed April 2018].

Shoemaker, R., n.d. *Surviving Mold.* [Online]
Available at: http://www.survivingmold.com/diagnosis
[Accessed April 2018].

University of Massachusetts Medical School, n.d. *Center for Mindfulness.* [Online]
Available at:
https://www.umassmed.edu/cfm/mindfulness-based-programs/mbsr-courses/about-mbsr/history-of-mbsr/
[Accessed April 2018].

Weil, A., n.d. *Dr Weil.* [Online]
Available at: https://www.drweil.com/videos-features/videos/breathing-exercises-4-7-8-breath/
[Accessed April 2018].

Wilson, V., 2016. *Balanced Women's Blog.* [Online]
Available at: http://balancedwomensblog.com/emotional-energy-centers/
[Accessed April 2018].

Resources

Section 4 - Wrestling with feeling ill

Dr Ian Gawler's history with cancer:
https://iangawler.com/about-drs-ian-and-ruth-gawler/#history

Cumulative Childhood Stress and Autoimmune Diseases in Adults:
https://www.ncbi.nlm.nih.gov/pmc/articles/PMC3318917/

Section 5 - Explore the road to here

Brad Yates – EFT Guru:
https://www.youtube.com/eftwizard

Lists of emotions for your reference:

http://positiveemotionslist.com/

http://negativeemotionslist.com/

Role of Physical Environment Summary

QUALITY OF AIR	QUALITY OF FOOD
Oxygen is pivotal in the functioning of your immune system. So, plenty of fresh air is required. Negative ions found concentrated near moving water increase levels of your happy hormone.	Source organic locally grown food. This includes fresh produce, animal and vegetable proteins, milk products etc. If in doubt consult 'dirty dozen' and 'clean fifteen' lists.
NOISE LEVEL	CHEMICAL FREE PRODUCTS
Noise exposure can have a negative influence on your well-being. It may increase your level of stress, which in turn can lead to a raised heart rate and blood pressure.	Your skin is the largest organ in the body and what we apply is absorbed into the bloodstream. Be an avid label reader and avoid anything with numbers and names you don't recognise

Starter list of Toxic Chemicals

Here is a starter list of toxic chemicals to watch out for and avoid.

Toxic Chemical	Found in
Parabens	Cosmetics, body wash, deodorant, shampoo, cleanser, foods, pharmaceutical products
Synthetic colours	Drugs, cosmetics and foods
Fragrance	Perfume, cologne, conditioner, shampoo, body wash, moisturiser
Phthalates	Deodorant, perfume, cologne, hair spray, moisturiser
Triclosan	Toothpaste, antibacterial soap, deodorant
Sodium lauryl sulphate (SLS) / Sodium laureth sulphate (SLES)	Shampoo, body wash, cleanser, cosmetics, acne treatments
Formaldehyde	Nail polish, body wash, conditioner, shampoo, cleansers, eye shadow, nail polish treatments
Toluene	Nail polish, nail treatments, hair colour, bleaching products

Toxic Chemical	Found in
Propylene glycol	Moisturiser, sunscreen, cosmetics, conditioner, shampoo, hair spray
PEG/Ceteareth/Polyethylene compounds	Cosmetics, toothpaste, pharmaceuticals, foods
BPH and BPA	Plastic food containers, lining of cans

USA Data for pesticides and chemicals

On the *Environment Working Group* (EWG) website you will find the *Dirty Dozen* and extended list of foods with pesticide residue and the *Clean Fifteen* list as a guide if you can't source organic - https://www.ewg.org/foodnews/

Note: Unless the corn and papaya are labelled organic I would recommend you avoid it, given your immune system is likely compromised already

Skin Deep Database by EWG - http://www.ewg.org/skindeep/top-tips-for-safer-products/#.WqRxMChubMU

Peer reviewed research articles highlighting the impact of pesticides on dis-ease

https://www.ncbi.nlm.nih.gov/pmc/articles/PMC3945755/

https://www.ncbi.nlm.nih.gov/pmc/articles/PMC5089872/

https://www.ncbi.nlm.nih.gov/pmc/articles/PMC4782969/

Section 6 – Experience of normalising the abnormal

MySymptoms Food Diary and Symptom Tracker: http://skygazerlabs.com/wp/

Section 7 - Journey through the medical system

Functional and Integrative Practitioners Insights

Some of the Functional and Integrative practitioners that I follow and gain insights from are:

Andrea Beaman - https://andreabeaman.com/

Dr Ben Lynch - https://www.drbenlynch.com/articles/

Dr Chris Kresser - https://chriskresser.com/articles/

Dr Deanna Minich - http://deannaminich.com/dr-deanna-minich-blog/

Dr Dan Khalish - https://kalishinstitute.com/blog/

Dr David Perlmutter - https://www.drperlmutter.com/blog/

Dr Frank Lipman - https://www.bewell.com/blog/

Dr Jeffrey Bland - http://jeffreybland.com/articles/

Dr Josh Axe - https://draxe.com/

Dr Mark Hyman - http://drhyman.com/blog/

Dr Marty Ross - http://www.treatlyme.net/treat-lyme-book/category/free/

Dr Natasha Campbell-McBride - http://www.doctor-natasha.com/

Dr Ritchie Shoemaker - http://www.survivingmold.com/news/

Dr Todd Le Pine - https://drlepine.com/blog/

Dr Tom O'Bryan - http://thedr.com/

Sites for finding a Functional Medicine Doctor

A sample of links to member or alumni-based sites for functional medicine doctors:

- Primal Docs - https://re-findhealth.com/members/
- Functional Medicine University - www.functionalmedicinedoctors.com
- The Institute of Functional Medicine (IFM) doctor locator - https://www.ifm.org/find-a-practitioner/

Section 8 - Finding your support crew

Morning Pages by Julia Cameron -
http://juliacameronlive.com/basic-tools/morning-pages/

Patti Villalobos Coaching: http://www.pattivillalobos.com

Section 9 - Your body - your vehicle for life

Nourish Well

FREE video series - www.livingfabulously.com/resources

- Hassle free Gluten free
- Live the Sweet life, Sugar free
- Healthy me Dairy free

Move More

Lauren Gelman article:

http://www.rd.com/health/fitness/6-ways-exercise-makes-
your-brain-better/

Rest and Recover

Self-paced Sleep Fabulously program:
http://bit.ly/sleepfabulously

Section 10 - Your mind - a playground for thoughts

Dr Andrew Weil demonstrating the 4-7-8 breath: https://www.drweil.com/videos-features/videos/breathing-exercises-4-7-8-breath/

Guru Nischan demonstrating Alternate Nostril Breathing: https://youtu.be/0uBssStT5yQ?t=3m33s

Download your Calm and Collected audio: https://www.livingfabulously.com/calm-and-collected

Mindfulness Based Stress Reduction free course: https://palousemindfulness.com/

Podcast with Kathy Gruver: http://bit.ly/Ep061-DrKathyGruver

Tips to avoid anxiety by Petrea King: https://wendymak.com/top-ten-tips-avoid-anxiety-guest-blogger-petrea-king/

Quest for Life Foundation: http://www.questforlife.com.au/residential-programs

Insight Timer App: https://insighttimer.com/

Section 11 - Your soul - the essence guiding you

Tracy Otsuka: https://www.coreintelligenceagency.com/

Tools for refreshing your values

What are your values from Mindtools:
https://youtu.be/Kz__qGJmTMY

Life values inventory assessment and recommendations:
http://www.lifevaluesinventory.org/

ACCOUNTABILITY
WITH A PEER GROUP
WHO CHEER YOU ON

ONLINE
BOOK CLUB

Would you like to be surrounded by people who understand how challenging the simplest things can be?

The ONLINE BOOK CLUB is to read and implement the strategies from 'Hope in a Dark Tunnel' with people who get you. The right level of support providing you with the accountability, hope and resilience to walk your path with courage.

Register your interest by sending an email to hello@livingfabulously.com

www.ingramcontent.com/pod-product-compliance
Lightning Source LLC
Chambersburg PA
CBHW032145020426
42334CB00016B/1232